The Only Herbal Remedies Book You'll Ever Need

How to Naturally Improve Your Health with Powerful Healing Herbs and 300+ Simple and Effective Plant Remedies

Aiyana Lewis

Table of Contents

Part I

~

Introduction to Herbal Medicine

Introduction

The western medical system has lost sight of the valuable knowledge passed down to us by our indigenous ancestors, who valued their health and wellness through natural means. This manuscript has been produced to provide comprehensive information about the secrets of natural healing through plants, herbs, and other means of medicine used by Native American traditional healers.

Anthropologists have identified over 1,300 species of medicinal plants that were used by Native Americans. Another 400 species are reported to have been used occasionally.

The word *herbal* refers to the fact that many native medicinal plants grew in or near water. The following were used by Native Americans:

Common Herbs: The most common herbs were those found everywhere around us, such as cedar bark, juniper berries, sumac leaves and roots, sarsaparilla root, willow bark, and several others. These were usually used for pain relief and fevers. Some herbs were used as food, such as the wild potato and sunflower seeds.

Sweet Herbs: Most sweet edible herbs were the root of a plant, such as rhubarb, sassafras, or wild ginger. They were not commonly used for medicinal purposes but were used as a tasty treat.

Felled Herbs: A plant that was growing on the forest floor would be felled and used for medicinal purposes. These would include dandelion leaves and roots, pine needles, burdock root, mints, and alfalfa leaves, which are rich in iron. Most of these plants grow in damp climates where they are hunted down by bears and other animals, and their use is usually intended to please the spirits.

Freshwater: Freshwater plants were used primarily to treat burns, rheumatism, and skin conditions. As ducks, fishes depend on these plants, and it is clear that the medicine was meant for them too. The most common of these are cattail roots, wild rice, and other plants like arrowroot and sago.

Aquatic Herbs: Plants found in or near the water were also used as medicine. These included sumac leaves (known as "suma"), blue lily stems (also called "water lily"), pondweed (ga-go-go) leaves, eelgrass leaves, and greenbrier roots. These were all considered good for treating burns and ulcers.

One report stated that 90% of the plants used by Native Americans were found in the eastern part of what is now the United States. This would include sagebrush, cactus, cottonwood bark, wild raspberry leaves, and wild plum fruit—which were all widely used for medicinal purposes.

In addition to herbal remedies, native people also made use of bones, stones, and clay. Many such charms have been found in graves or other time-tested locations where an object was used to help a person in some way or another.

Many of these medicinal charms have been found in gravesites and were associated with the dead. Beads, earrings, animal bones, and other objects that were shaped into a certain form were used to represent the spirits. The spirit world was believed to be full of benevolent forces who would watch over the deceased for all eternity because they had been good people in life. The spirit world was also thought of as a possible haven for those who died at an early age or in battle. Many tribes expressed this through a belief that warriors who died went to some kind of heaven, and their spirits protected their tribes from enemies, illness, and other misfortunes.

Your Journey to A Completely Healthy Life

Know Before You Make a Decision

For the many people that try out Native medicines without success, it is mostly because of the lack of knowledge. People are very much emotional about things, jumping to conclusions and following the crowd, just because of some testimonial.

Native American medicines have been used for years. Even though its effects may not be as serious as they were thousands of years ago due to poor data keeping, but people have testified to its potency. Then, you can't just jump on the bandwagon. You need to get yourself educated first before taking any native medicine.

Get a Diagnosis

The first thing you want to do is to find out about your disease. You want to do as many tests as required so that you'll know exactly what is wrong or right with you. You want to know everything as much as you can. This is why you have to work very closely with your doctor so that there will be some monitoring as you embark on this journey into healing by nature. Once you understand what you're dealing with, you can now move to the next stage.

Understand your ailment and healing options. Most people that seek native medicine have in mind that because it is natural, it is far better than orthodox medicine. While this may be true for some medical issues, it may not be true for all. For example, there are situations or health problems that will certainly require medical surgery before it will go. There are no alternatives. If you are in this type of situation, it will do you good to consider surgery first.

Understanding your ailment also ensures that errors are limited or cut down to zero. No matter how determined you think you are, the nature of your ailment will always be the major determinant to know if it is something you should wholly subject to treatment through herbs.

Do Research

In addition to working with your doctor, you should also try and do your own research about what is wrong with you. This is even more important for people who have been dealing with certain ailments for a very long time.

Your research should be on the causes, triggers, and prevention options for your ailment. If your doctor thinks that you should try conventional medicine first, you can go on with it as long as you can afford it. If not, you still need to discuss with your doctor about herbals—and how you are going to use them the right way.

Who Should Consider Native American Medicine?

There are certain groups of people who should consider Native American medicines more. Of course, it is available for all, but these people should take it even more seriously as it could be a very lasting solution to their problems.

You've Tried Conventional Medicine without Changes

Evidence has shown that some people suffering from seemingly minor ailments had struggled with it for years, without any proper results. For example, many people have reported dealing with insomnia, migraine, or headaches for years without finding a solution after taking plenty of pills. If you fall into this category, it is important that you consider alternative medicine like Native American medicine. You need to discuss with your doctor about options before moving on to the alternative way.

You're Tired of Taking Pills

Some people have taken pills so much that it has become a mental burden.

Yes, if you find solid information about natural remedies, it is normal to feel that you want to get rid of the chemicals. Native medicine offers you the opportunity to try out nature in its unprocessed form. Our body contains similar elements that are available in nature. This makes it safe and acceptable for our internal organs.

You Hate Drug Side Effects

Many conventional medicines have side effects that might even be worse than the ailment itself. Some people have endured sleepless nights, skin rash, stomach upset, headaches, nausea, vomiting, itching, etc, just because they want to get a cure. Most herbs don't have serious side effects unless you don't take them in moderation. In fact, there are herbs that can help you overcome some of the side effects caused by the use of conventional medicine.

You Want a Combination

Sometimes your prescriptions may be working perfectly, but you still want to include natural herbs. You need to talk to your doctor and see how this works out. Self-medication in any form is dangerous. Not to talk of herbs that you have no idea of what they contain. Your doctor will be able to guide you in the kind of herbs you can take. They will also guide you on how to make it work with your pills. Many people have experienced faster recovery, fewer drug side effects, and better drug assimilation when they did it right.

You Want to Save Money

Conventional medicine is expensive. Perhaps this is among the reasons why many people want to try out alternative medicines, which can provide the same results with a smaller bill. Understandably, alternative medicine is cheaper because it is made from nature. The raw materials are derived from plants, trees, leaves, and roots that cost little to nothing to get.

The manufacturing and processing are also very easy, and most times, the herbs come with their own natural preservatives, so they don't get spoiled for a very long time. Alternative medicine can save you a lot of money, and at the same time, they give you even more relief compared to what conventional medicine can do for you.

You Want to Try out New Things

If you have been using pills all your life for minor ailments, like headaches, pain, sore throat, and cold, it is a great thing for anyone to try out. You'll be doing some exciting experiments with your body, and you will be able to measure the difference between both methods. Trying out alternative medicine will also help you discover new things about your body. The more new things you discover about yourself, the healthier you'll live—no doubt about that.

Medicinal Plants Used Daily by Native Americans

Butterbur ("Petasites")

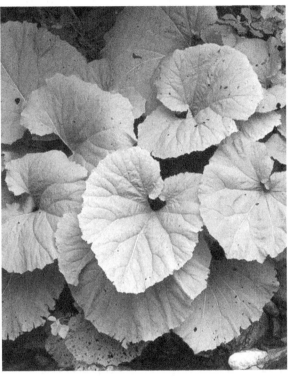

Butterbur, also known as "Petasites," is another medicinal herb found in the Pacific North West. It is a perennial plant with thick rhizomes that creep underground. It can also be identified by its leaves, which are rhubarb-like. Parts of this plant that are usable for medicinal purposes include the roots, leaves, and stems.

So, why is it ideal for treating headaches? The plant contains certain active substances called "petasin" and "isopetasin." These compounds dampen inflammation, which in turn reduces headaches and migraines.

It is found in parts of Europe, Asia, and the USA. It commonly grows in areas that are wet and marshy. You can also get it in forests that are damp and along streams.

Mullein ("Verbascum")

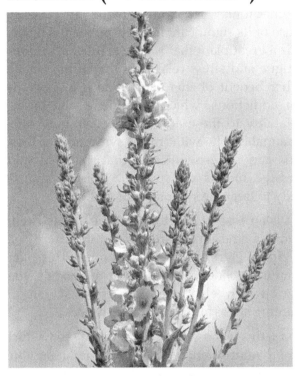

Mullein is a perennial plant that grows to around 3 meters tall. The leaves of this plant are soft, hairy, and arranged in a spiral manner. The flowers are yellow and appear atop the plant, giving it a unique appearance. The parts of this plant that are of medicinal value are leaves and flowers.

So, why is it good for treating nasal congestion? The plant contains tannin, which has astringent properties. What this means is that it brings about the contraction of cells and tissues. This helps reduce the inflammation, which in turn reduces the irritation caused by nasal congestion. This is why it is an effective remedy for nasal congestion. This plant is found in Europe, Asia, and the Americas. It is often spotted in areas such as fields and ditches. If you are having a hard time finding it, you can easily find it in most natural food stores.

Oat Seed ("Avena sativa")

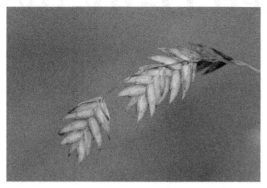

"Nervine tonic" is another name of oat seed because of its significant impacts on mental health. This is a great plant that is used to treat symptoms of fatigue and stress related to the brain's health. Another benefit of this plant is to use it against many addictions, which are due to the brain's adaptability to these addictions, such as nicotine and cannabis. The withdrawal symptoms of these plants can be so intense that agitated and aggressive moods can prevail. It is a fantastic remedy to treat the symptoms of addiction.

Stress is an essential factor that is associated with the brain's stress and fatigue, and the use of oat seed effectively treats these symptoms. This plant has fantastic benefits of restoring the body's vital energy, which also plays an essential role in preventing stress and mood disturbances.

Avena sativa is the generic name of oat seed, which is used to nourish and improve the human nervous system. Anxiety, impaired sleep, and decreased sexual performance, which are the secondary impacts of stress, can also be treated directly by using oat seeds regularly. This plant has superior benefits over many other herbs because of having an abundant supply of vitamins and minerals, which are highly crucial for the proper performance of the nervous system.

Adrenal stress can also be treated by using oat seeds in these two types of formulations.

Green Tea ("Camellia sinensis")

Tea is well known and probably the most consumed beverage in the world.

The use of this herb for medicinal purposes is well known and has a strong research background.

Black tea requires the essential and partial fermentation process of the tea leaves. However, green tea doesn't require these kinds of fermentation and can be produced through the process of steaming the leaves.

This process reduces the oxidation capacities of enzymes present in tea leaves, and the preservation of polyphenol is achieved through this process. It is interesting to know that polyphenols belong to a family of flavonoids that represent 30–40% of the total weight in dried green tea leaves.

Camellia sinensis is a known name for dried and unfermented green tea leaves. It has the property to reduce bacterial and viral activities in the body. It is also essential in lowering down the increased concentration of lipids in the blood. The potency of green tea to lower down the blood cholesterol level is excellent, and thus it is a beverage of choice to reduce some extra pounds from the body. It is a potent anti-lipidemic agent. Its antioxidant benefits make it a perfect choice to detoxify the liver, kidneys, intestine, stomach, and skin. Its detoxifying and lipid-lowering benefits make it a perfect choice as a natural healer. The scientific base behind green tea is solid, and it is used in traditional as well as modern medicine as a natural source to treat many common illnesses of the human body. It is a super herb in holism, and the benefits of this herb are beyond the capacity of this essential book on holism.

Devil's Club ("Oplopanax horridus")

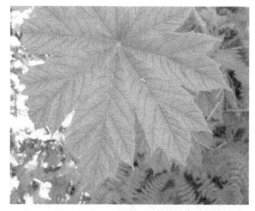

This plant belongs to the ginseng family, and botanically, it is considered in the "Araliaceae family." Another name implied to this plant is devil's stick or devil's walking cane. Its roots leave as well as stem are used for herbal medicinal purposes in herbalism.

It should not be confused with the devil's claw, which is a plant grown in hot deserts.

This plant is widely produced in the northwest of America. It also contains many attributes of the ginseng family, which is essential to treat diabetes. It helps in curing insulin resistance. It also helps in lowering increased cholesterol levels in the blood.

The most significant benefit of this herb is its use in weight loss and weight management coach—who knows its herbal impact, can help his/her client to reduce some extra pounds in a natural and effective manner. This plant is really a blessing for diabetic patients because it helps in increasing the blood insulin levels and in reducing the blood glucose spike after meals, which can be dangerous for pre-diabetics and full-blown diabetic patients.

Its anti-inflammatory and antioxidant nature helps in the recovery of cancer patients because it helps in reducing the weight and extra fat in cancer patients, which is caused by stress. Cancer patients also possess poor insulin tolerance, and thus, it helps in this regard as well.

Alpha-Lipoic Acid ("S or R-Lipoic Acid")

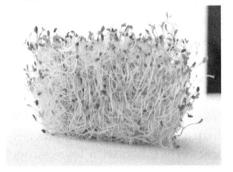

It is also an essential supplement that is widely used in herbalism to cure many disorders and to prevent many diseases. Carrots, yams, and beef, as well as another type of red meat, are rich in alpha-lipoic acid. It has significant impacts on the energy supply of the body called "ATP." It also has global effects on the body and can benefit nearly every organ and system of the body, including skin, liver, kidney, heart, and pancreas. It also has many antioxidant benefits, which makes it fit for everyday use.

In the body's cells, alpha-lipoic acid contributes to enhancing the power of power grid units called "mitochondria." It has been proved in cadaveric studies that alpha-lipoic acid is highly essential in treating age-related changes in the brain. It is a significant health supplement for patients with Parkinson's and Alzheimer's diseases.

It is a very natural type of COX-2 inhibitor, which is used as an anti-inflammatory and pain killer agent in many allopathic drugs. It is also very rich in glutathione and vitamin C. All these characteristics make it a perfect supplement for daily use.

In my practice and experience, my top 5 herb selections tend to cover all my home-healing bases time and time again. Whether it relates to aches, cramps, nerves, or bruises—almost anything, really—I can usually turn to one of my fabulous five without a second thought. All their effects are well-studied, trusted, and even versatile and far-reaching, covering a wide variety of ailments, troubles, and injuries. With some luck and practice, I'm sure they'll become your trusted allies, too!

But once in a while, you need another support herb (or two!) to cover your tail. Maybe one of this top 5 just isn't doing the trick and needs a helping herb to go the extra mile. That or you've run out your favorite go-to herb in your herbal cabinet, cupboard, or growing at-home apothecary.

Alfalfa ("Medicago sativa")

A digestive cleanser, tonic, and nutritious food and medicine.

Enjoy Alfalfa sprouts? Both studies and traditional medicine hold that alfalfa can have healing effects that combat cancer and digestive ailments. Use Alfalfa by eating it as sprouts or raw leaves in meals, or use fresh leaves in a thick infusion every day. Alfalfa is typically available as an over-the-counter supplement as well.

Alfalfa is a very cleansing digestive detoxifier for the gut. The research observed alfalfa binds to carcinogens in the colon. European studies suggest regular consumption of alfalfa helps in lowering cholesterol.

Alfalfa leaves are a significant source of vitamin K, potassium, iron, zinc, and protein (as well as vitamin A, B1, B6, C, and E.)

Never consume alfalfa seeds, especially in high amounts daily, as they will lead to developing a blood clotting disorder.

Arnica ("Arnica montana")

A sunny healer for bruises, muscle aches, sprains, and arthritis.

Use the dried flower heads in oils, salves, or tinctures for applying to the skin where muscles, bones, or joints are sore. Or, visit your local natural food or medicine section—arnica creams and ointments tend to be popular and plenty!

Applying arnica relieves pain and swelling greatly in bruises, contusions, or muscular injuries where the skin is not open. This is due to observed sesquiterpene lactones thought to activate and intensely fight inflammation.

Teas, tisanes, or liniments (in tincture or vinegar form) can be applied to areas in need of musculoskeletal pain relief. The flower heads can also be heated and bruised as a poultice.

Never take Arnica internally or put the product on open skin, such as wounds or burns. It can cause heart and respiratory problems if absorbed into the bloodstream.

Black Haw ("Viburnum prunifolium")

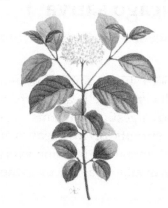

This beautiful bush—with bright red berries and cream-colored flowers—is a cornerstone favorite in United States Southern herbalism. It was once used for all sorts of women's health issues by Native Americans—even for childbirth, miscarriage, and labor. Now, it has settled into the comfortable role of allaying uterine cramps that accompany menstruation—but anyone, man or woman, can enjoy its ability to take away intestinal or stomach cramps as well.

A compound in the roots and stems called "scopoletin" works to soothe spasms in smooth muscles, whether found in the digestive tract or uterus. It also works on the smooth muscle in the trachea, making black haw beneficial for asthma symptoms and attacks.

Black haw should not be used in women who are pregnant, children under 16, or those with aspirin allergies.

Black Cohosh ("Actaea racemose")

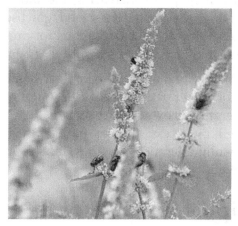

It is a nature's healing hormonal resource for women, and it is native to North America. This stunning plant (once used for snakebites in native herbalism) has become an important herbal medicine for women today. It contains compounds called "phytoestrogens," which mimic estrogen and fit perfectly in female hormone receptors.

Some herbalists say that black cohosh is good for women with menstrual problems. More precisely, it is more relieving for women with low estrogen levels, especially women in menopause. It can provide a natural hormone replacement therapy but check with your physician.

Some menstrual issues are, in fact, due to low estrogen. If you have PCOS (polycystic ovarian syndrome), adult acne issues, and/or irregular menses, consider getting your hormone levels checked and trying black cohosh.

Avoid it if you are pregnant, and make sure you are taking Black Cohosh, not Blue Cohosh, which can be dangerous. Avoid taking it if you have liver disease.

Part II

~

Secrets of Herbal Medicine

Native American Medicine

Native American medicine is a holistic approach to healing that incorporates the usage of certain plants and animals, as well as breathing techniques. In this chapter, we will discuss the various remedies Native Americans would use for healing and how these remedies have been adapted for modern society today.

In spite of its wide-ranging popularity in many Native American tribes, the use of these medicines is relatively unknown in contemporary Western culture. That's because Western doctors generally work with a system that relies on surgery or medications as their primary treatments—both methods can adversely affect your health if overused.

Native American Beliefs on Religion and Healing

Beliefs on religion and healing vary from culture to culture, but some Native American beliefs are similar. In general, the Creator created all things in the beginning. All men/women have a soul that is eternal and has been with them since birth. The Creator made humans equal and stated that some people would be born pure and others would carry a curse from one of their ancestors. When first sinned, the Creator took away human's immortality and had them die again until they had placed their trust in him again.

As per Native American beliefs on religion and healing, people must free themselves from evil spirits (usually via ceremony) or risk being punished by those spirits throughout life. Evil spirits, or ghosts, are believed to be the cause of all sicknesses in Native American culture. When an evil spirit is released from a person's body through the ceremony, that person is healed. The people of the tribe believe they are continuing the cycle of life by performing ceremonies.

Shamans are healers who have been chosen to help heal members of their tribe who may be ill. They are known in a variety of ways, including those using herbs and medicinal plants, but many practices also include rituals and magic. The more magical aspects of Native American beliefs on religion and healing often include contact with animal spirits and other good spiritual forces via dreams or visions. If there is something physically wrong with a person, shamans use medicinal plants to heal them.

Treatment Approach

The Native American Indians practiced a type of medicine that was handed down from generation to generation. They combined many resources, including leaves, barks, roots, and minerals that helped them treat various ailments or heal from an injury. There were specific plants for treating specific conditions, and the tribes would often trade with each other in order to obtain the right plants for their needs. Sometimes they would use parts of animals as well as insects to create a healing product. The natives had studied the effects of these substances and knew what was fatal when ingested or not toxic when used externally on wounds and bodily injuries or illnesses.

Theories and Meaning of the Four Directions

Native Americans believe that there are four directions in life, each with its own special significance. The North is the direction of the sky, and it is associated with direction, wisdom, power, and leadership. The East directs us towards our future and growth, which symbolizes knowledge, intellect, and understanding. The South is where the Earth resides—it's this direction that embodies balance or harmony. And lastly, we have the west, which represents a return to family and relatives as well as a return to your roots or origins—home.

Native American Medicine and the Four Directions

These four directions are represented by four colors: The North is white, the East is red, the South is Blue, and the West is black.

In ancient Native America, the four colors represented the directions and their corresponding elements. For example, yellow was seen as a spiritual color that symbolized the Earth, but it also represented all of creation in its infinite beginnings and ends. "Yellow" was thought to be "fullness of life." Blue was also highly regarded, as it symbolized mental ability and creativity, but can mean other things too; it can represent water or sky, so it has a certain "ethereal" quality. Blue is also a spiritual color, and it represents the "Great Spirit" or "Creator."

"Orange" was used in Native American paintings and pottery to represent "the color of fire" or "the color of the sun." Orange is associated with health, fertility, energy, and warmth. It is also thought of as "golden," which represents the union of Heaven and Earth. Red was thought to be a healing color representing life, but it has many other meanings, too. Red can mean danger and war, or it can mean happiness, love, and joy. It usually symbolizes earth in its various stages; red can also be seen as a spiritual color representing God's presence on earth. It was also thought to be a powerful color for self-protection. White is also a spiritual color as it represents the purity of being and truth and as a means to purify ourselves of our "sins." However, white can also be seen as the color of God himself in nature, in dreams or in life—when we have no other choice but to let go.

Story of Herbs

Herbs are aromatic plants that are grown for their savory flavor, fragrance, and medicinal properties. They've been used for thousands of years to heal wounds and cure infections. Nowadays, they're also commonly found in the kitchen. While many herbs can be grown in a small pot on a windowsill, there is something to be said about harvesting them fresh from the wild or purchasing them from a local farm stand during warmer months.

Herbs in the Kitchen

Experiment with a variety of herbs to find out which ones you like the best. Lavender, mint, chamomile, lemon balm, and rosemary are some popular choices that hold their flavor even after being dried. Sage is another herb that can be used in a multitude of dishes and is traditionally used to rub on poultry or roast before cooking to add flavor. Experiment with fresh herbs by adding them to sauces for meats or mixing them into potato salad for a flavorful twist.

Dried herbs work best with soups and stews or when they're added near the end of the cooking process, such as with roasts or casseroles. Some herbs, such as thyme and rosemary, are best when fresh rather than dried. Thyme can be used in a variety of dishes, including stews, soups, and meatloaf, as well as in herb butter. Rosemary is commonly used to season everything from roast chicken to sides of potatoes or greens.

Herbal Teas for Healing Purposes

Many herbs can be made into teas to soothe illness or even treat certain medical conditions. Chamomile is a popular tea that is known to help with insomnia, while peppermint aids digestion (it can also help relieve headaches and stomach pains). Mint can also be used in baked goods like cookies for an extra layer of flavor. Ginger tea has been used to help with nausea, and a cheery lemon-mint combination is effective in clearing a stuffy nose. Finally, chamomile can be made into a soothing tea and taken as needed.

Herbal Infused Oils

Infused oils can be made with fresh herbs or dried. Mint, sage, rosemary, thyme, oregano, and curry are some of the most popular ones to use for cooking. They can also be used in marinades or herbal baths for added flavors. These blends add an extra layer of flavor to dishes while adding nourishment to your diet as well as your body.

When making your own infused oils, be sure to use the best quality extra-virgin olive oil you can afford. Add dried herbs to warm oil in a saucepan over low heat, and allow it to sit for a few hours or overnight. Strain out the herbs using a cheesecloth before storing. The longer you let them sit, the stronger the flavor will be.

Herbs are an important part of a healthy diet. Adding fresh herbs can be an easy way to sneak more nutrients into your daily meals without tasting like medicine. They also serve as natural remedies for ailments such as headaches, allergies, and indigestion, if taken in liquid form or infused into foods like butter or vinegar.

Different Herbal Healing Systems

Throughout the globe, the use of herbs in different healing systems ("herb lore" or origins and historical significance) is rooted in various religious beliefs. In some cultures, these medicinal plants are ascribed supernatural abilities to heal or ward off evil. Ayurveda uses more than two dozen plants for their therapeutic value. Many of these herbs were originally used to treat snakebite, which makes sense, given that snakes are universally associated with evil and violence.

According to the Western herbalism system—based on ancient Greek medicine—a plant could have either a hot or cold effect on the body and was also believed to have other properties, such as moistening or drying effects. For example, a plant that caused sweating was thought to be cold and dry. Inversely, a plant that caused dryness and itching would be hot and dry. This can be found in the work of authors such as Pliny the Elder (AD 23–79). The "Kleinia" was an early species of plant discovered in Greece by Aristotle in 335 BC; it is still used today as herbal medicine.

The herbal medicine tradition has been studied through history—particularly with respect to alchemical symbolism and magical qualities ascribed to plants by early historians, such as Aelian, Dioscorides, Pliny the Elder, or Tertullian. The tradition was also used for the translation of texts, as a means for research or just as a means for studying the properties and uses of herbs.

According to modern herbal medicine, there are around 200,000 plant species. Herbalism is also practiced in various forms by diverse groups of people.

There are various forms of herbalism practiced around the world that have developed over time and which vary greatly based on ethnic groups and cultures. In areas where Western medicine predominates, it tends to take the form of pharmacopeia. The Indigenous Peoples of Amazonia and their neighbors use herbalism mainly as supportive measures in traditional healing practices.

Different herbal healing systems have different approaches to their history and healing modalities. Some cultures have developed a complex relationship with herbs, which has led to a long tradition of herbal medicine. In many traditional societies, herbs and other plants were and continue to be valued for their medicinal properties as well as for the positive effects they have on the spiritual lives of people in particular communities.

In contrast, the Western approach is based mostly on pharmacology and medical practice. It is common in Westernized cultures to only consider plants that are sold in the pharmacy or supermarket as medicinal or useful for certain conditions. Herbalism may be dismissed outright because it is viewed as irrational, although religious texts from various faiths continue to recognize its importance.

A common viewpoint in the West is that herbs and other plants are "simply" plants. Therefore, they do not have an intrinsic value—unlike animals, which may be more highly regarded due to their generally greater ability to experience pleasure or pain. Herbalists often reject this view.

The Use of Herbs in Ancient Religions

The use of herbs in ancient religions is one of the many ways that mankind has attempted to understand and control their world. The earliest evidence we have for this activity comes from the remains of plant material found in archaeological sites, but it is likely that people have been using herbs throughout ancient history for various reasons.

The medical text "Sushruta Samhita" contains one of the first known references to the medicinal use of plants. Written in Sanskrit, this chapter contains descriptions and drawings of 657 preparations, as well as information about when they should be used and how they should be prepared. This text has been dated to around the 8th century BCE (medieval India).

The famous "Perseus" statue is presumed to have been made in approximately 100 BCE from a gold-coated bronze alloy containing malachite—which is an extract from the root of a "Malvaceae" (mallow) plant. The statue depicts the Greek divine hero Perseus holding up ahead, which is said to be that of Medusa. This creature was once thought to be immortal but is now known to be capable of being killed by a swift blow with an arrow by its reflection in the eyes. The head would turn whoever looked upon it into stone, and they would be unable to turn back until someone removed the head. In the story, Perseus used an obsidian (a volcanic glass) sword to kill Medusa.

An international group of scientists have extracted DNA from a skull dating back to between 12,000 and 7,000 years old and have discovered that this skull is closely related to the one belonging to a Northern European woman who lived around 4,400 years ago. This means that people were already using plants in Eurasia at least 3,500 years before they were used in the Americas.

"Sushruta Samhita" is a medical text, and the use of herbs in ancient religions is one of the many ways that mankind has attempted to understand and control their world. The earliest evidence we have for this activity comes from the remains of plant material found in archaeological sites, but it is likely that people have been using herbs throughout ancient history for various reasons.

Ancient religions often gave equal value to all-natural products. Herbs were often used in religious ceremonies—both to heal and to treat disease and as an offering to spirits or gods. Some examples of this are:

"The Carved Goddess," found in Cyprus, is dated around 1,500 BCE, though its original purpose is unknown. It is carved in greenstone and is thought by some to represent a female figure. It has also been suggested to be a fertility symbol, and it has been suggested that it may have possible medicinal uses.

A Short History of Plants as Medicines

Plants have been used for medicinal purposes for as long as humans have inhabited earth. The earliest known evidence for the use of plants in healing dates back to over 10,000 BC and can be found in the form of a petroglyph in an area known today as Switzerland. The petroglyph illustrates a man facing what is thought to be a banyan tree, of which trunk has nine crowns with five leaves sprouting from each of them, while the surrounding text reads "WHEN THE WIND BLOWS…," it is thought to indicate that this plant has powerful medicinal properties. This discovery suggests that in the far reaches of time, there was already some knowledge of the medicinal properties of plants.

Humans have long been aware of and benefited from the healing powers of plants. The ancient Egyptians used different plants to heal many ailments and diseases, from toothaches to depression. In fact, modern-day aspirin is still made in a similar fashion—by grinding willow bark and extracting salicylic acid from it. Many other cultures also have a history of using plants as medicine, with many civilizations contributing to its development and understanding over time. One of the most famous civilizations that did this was the Aztecs, who used many different plant species to cure diseases and ailments. The Aztecs, for example, used the leaves of the maguey plant to make pulque (a fermented drink). It is thought that they also used it to make an ointment for treating wounds and inflammation. Apparently, Mexican Indians have been using this herbal medicine for centuries. Many other cultures of the world also knew about and utilized indigenous medicinal plants, but it was not until recently that western countries started taking an interest in their benefits.

Herbal Preparations

Using Fresh Plants — Harvesting and Drying

- **Compressed Herbs:** Dry the herbs with a dehydrator.
- **Freezing Herbs:** Use a sealable plastic bag and freezer.
- **Dried Herb Powder:** Mix the herbs with a food processor or coffee grinder. (You can also use it in herbal tea mixes. When blended together, it is called an "iced tea mix." You can purchase dried herb powder at many health food stores or online.)
- **Tinctures:** Add 25% alcohol to the mixture and stir well, then add 1 tablespoon of this tincture to 2 tablespoons of water before drinking or putting it into herbal teas.
- **Herbal Tea:** Making your own herbal tea is quick and easy. (It is best to steep the herbs in boiling water for at least ten minutes, but most herbs can be prepared in a few minutes or overnight.)
  (Another herb-rich beverage is "rosehip tea," which people especially drink when they are feeling in the weather. It's also delicious iced.)
- **Infusions:** Place 1 teaspoon of dried herb into a cup of hot water and leave it for 5–10 minutes to let the herb's healing properties seep through. Remove from the heat and allow the liquids to cool down before drinking.
  Soak 1 teaspoon of dried herb in hot water for 5–10 minutes. Soak in cold water for 20 minutes. Mix with 1 teaspoon of honey or stevia. Drink as is or steep for 10 minutes and add as desired to herbal tea.
- **Jams and Jellies:** 1 cup of dried herbs yields about 10–15 servings — a little goes a long way, so don't add too much! The simplest way to make jam is by combining 1 cup of fresh herbs with 2 cups of tepid water, bringing it to a boil, and stirring constantly until the mixture thickens (about 30–45 minutes). Adding a little honey or sugar will preserve the jam.
- **Dill Pickles:** Place 6 tablespoons of dried dill weed into 2 cups of boiling water and steep for 10 minutes. Strain the mixture, adding 2 sprigs of fresh dill to the liquid, and pour it into a clean jar with 1 cup of cucumbers cut up into pieces (fresh or peeled). Pour 3 cups of vinegar over the cucumbers and seal. The pickles can be eaten immediately but are best if left in a cool, dark place for about 2 weeks before serving.
- **Herbal Extract Tincture:** Add alcohol to the herbs and letting it infuse for no less than two weeks to extract maximum aroma and flavor properties.

Infusions

Infusions are water-based liquids to which medicinal plants or plant parts have been added. Infusions are made by steeping an ingredient, such as leaves, flowers, or roots, in boiled water for a given time period. The resulting liquid is then strained and consumed either hot (usually) or cold.

Some common infusions you may be familiar with are peppermint tea and chamomile tea. Hot peppermint tea is one of the most popular drinks during winter to help soothe your throat and stomach aches, while chamomile tea aids in relaxation and sleep. Both of these teas are simple to make, but as you learn more about them, their recipes and procedures may seem daunting. This chapter will teach you the basic steps to making this type of tea, and in no time, you'll be ready to impress your friends with your pallet-perfected green tea!

Infusions are wonderful for people who wish to drink medicine without ingesting large amounts of active ingredients or even those who are allergic to specific plants or compounds, as this may occur in plants like black pepper berry.

Another great thing about infusions is that they can be made with decoctions, which have the same effect as infusions—they create a remedy derived from plants. Some people dislike the taste of decoctions; however, infusions can be much more appealing if they are going to be drunk as medicine in liquid form. Decoctions are made by simmering a soup or other dish with medicinal herbs for a set amount of time, which makes them very similar to infusions. Infusions are much easier to make and require fewer ingredients than a decoction does, making them the perfect beginner's project for those interested in learning how to make medicine at home!

In the history of herbs, there have been many types of infusions put to use. Infusions are used for everything from health care, beauty treatments, and even wayward cooking. They've been classified as either hot or cold ingredients and often either made by boiling water or in the sun. There are pros and cons when using this method—with each type having its own benefits and drawbacks to how they are administered.

The Pros of Using Infusions

There are many pros to using infusions, and they are put to use in many ways, but a few key areas stand out.

Herbal infusions are ones that contain herbs that have been boiled in a pot or glass jar with boiling water. Herbs can be infused for medicinal reasons, beautification, cooking, and often times infused with oil or alcohol for extraction purposes. If you'd like to learn how to make an herbal infusion, then keep reading.

The first pro is the fact that they're easily administered. This is great for someone who wants to use herbs in a short period of time without having to go through too many steps to prepare them. It's also very easy to store, and it is easy on the budget when you decide how much of a certain herb you want to use and buy easy—only what you'd need.

Another pro tip is that they're often made in large quantities and can last for a while. The longer it sits, the stronger it becomes, so be sure not to let time pass by as quickly as the infusion does!

The Cons of Using Infusions

There are cons when using infusions, but these are not enough reasons not to use them if they suit your needs. Some cons include not extracting the beneficial properties of certain herbs—like using peppermint for headaches, for example.

It's also hard to measure how much of each herb you're using when making an infusion, which is why many people opt to use multiple at a time instead of just one.

The last con is that they take a while to make and often require more than 1 step in order to prepare them. It's best if you use the same glass jar every time you want to make an infusion because it will keep the ingredients in place and allow for the most consistent blend or flavor without having any extra ingredients added.

Hot infusions are typically used to make teas, such as chamomile tea. These are typically milder teas that are usually ingested, as opposed to cold infusions, which are often only used externally. This is because hot water tends to release the volatile and aromatic oils of the herb more quickly than cold water infusions do.

Cold infusions are made by placing herbs (either whole or ground) in a container with water and letting it sit overnight. They work slower than hot infusions, but they can be stored at room temperature for extended periods of time without degrading or losing their potency, so they can be used in topical applications. These types of preparations have been shown to have stronger flavors and a higher content of coumarin. For this reason, they tend to be more effective at alleviating inflammation.

Deciding Between Hot and Cold Infusions

The major difference in infusions is the differences in the heat used to prep them. Basically, hot infusions are made with boiling water that turns into steam and is then inhaled by a person's nose or from their mouth as they'd drink the infusion directly out of the pot. This allows for much better absorption of vitamins and minerals into a person's body. On the other hand, cold infusions are made with cold water, which doesn't boil over, so it won't turn into steam. Herbalists often keep both around for different occasions if they can't decide between hot and cold or have no idea what type they want to use.

Teas

Tea ("Camellia sinensis") is an evergreen plant. The leaves of the tea plant have been used in China for at least 2,000 years as a medicinal herb.

The therapeutic action of tea is attributed to the catechin polyphenols found in the leaf. Caffeine and other chemicals average only 2–15%.

Sun Teas

"Sun tea" or "sun brewing" is a type of herbal tea that uses water and sun instead of boiling water on the stove. The sun tea technique uses the heat of the sun and time to steep the herbs in water. The tea is commonly prepared in a jar with a small mesh bag containing the tea and a string attached to the lid so it can be hung in direct sunlight. Once brewed, sun tea has a dark amber color and tastes like a very strong green tea.

Decoction

A decoction is a boiled extraction of chemicals or herbal medicines from herbs or bones by boiling them in water on low heat for 10–60 minutes. The process is also called "Mo" or "Moxa" therapy, which is a Chinese word for "burning herbs." Mo is an important part of Traditional Chinese Medicine and is widely practiced in China today.

Juicing

Juicing is the process of extracting the phytochemicals from whole fruits and vegetables to create a juice. Juicing extracts more nutrients than just eating whole foods.

An often-used fruit or vegetable juice contains about 80% water — this part of the process is called dehydrating. The remaining portion of the fruit or vegetable juice consists of the chemicals, such as flavonoids, minerals, and vitamins that give a juice its color and flavor. The heart enzyme papain present in many fruits can also be used to extract these chemicals with a little more heat from the stove or electric juicer.

Fomentations

Fomentations are herbal dressings that are applied on top of an herbal compress to boost the herbs' effectiveness. Fomentations are made by soaking herbs in hot water, adding salt and other ingredients, and kneading until the mixture is soft. Decoctions or purées can also be made to form fomentation.

Poultice

A poultice, which is made by boiling herbs and applying them to the skin, usually in order to promote healing.

Poultices have been utilized for centuries in cultures all around the world as a natural healing therapy that can be applied to any area of your body, from shoulders to feet and everything in between. Poultices are mainly utilized to treat acute and chronic injuries (and skin infections), promote faster healing, and relieve pain.

Poultices can be made using a wide variety of ingredients, from plants to herbs, oils, clays, metals, and even animal feces. The ingredients are usually mixed together and applied directly to the skin; they are then covered with a bandage or cloth called a "poultice wrap."

Herbal Medicine

There are many different ideas about what herbal medicine is. Some people say it is a type of medicine that uses natural substances, such as herbs, leaves, and roots, to heal the body. Others define it as an approach to healing the body using these same natural substances in the form of teas, infusions, tinctures, and so on. Still, others may take a more spiritual approach by understanding herbal medicine to be an act of God through which people can come into harmony with nature's gifts. In general, terms though herbal medicine falls under two main categories, herbalism and phytotherapy or plant-based medicine, some people will use the categories together, and others may even consider that the two can be combined.

It is generally accepted that all of these terms encompass a wide variety of practices and solutions designed to help heal human ailments. Herbal remedies are commonly used for illnesses and certain conditions in general health, dieting, fitness, and disease prevention. They can be made up of natural substances such as plants, herbs or minerals (called plant-based medicines), which have been prepared in different forms (like teas, ointments, or poultices) to help provide a solution for an ailment.

Sources of Herbs

When considering sources of herbs, there are a few key items that should be taken into consideration. These items include, but are not limited to the following:

Herbs should be sourced from a clean environment. They should not have any type of chemical residue. Plants should be harvested when they are at their peak for quality and potency, and the plants which are harvested should be dried.

Herbs that have been sourced from an unclean environment may contain foreign particles or unwanted organisms. How can you tell if the herb is sourced from a clean environment? The leaves that have been cleaned and stripped off their stems can easily let you know. If the leaves are covered with grime or organisms, it is an indication that the herb was not harvested in an environment that is considered clean. The soil that has been growing the herb should also be clean. You can test this by extracting some of the dirt from where you will plant your herb and rubbing it on your face. If your face feels refreshed after rubbing, then you probably have a good source. However, if you feel like there is something wrong with the dirt, then you may want to find another location to grow your herbs.

Herbs should also contain no traces of chemicals from pesticides and other harmful substances that may be present in these plants when they are grown for consumption. They should not be sprayed with any type of pesticides or anything else that may hinder the overall quality of the plant. These chemicals will only weaken the overall strength of the herb, and they will not make good herbal medicine.

Herbs should be harvested when they are at their peak to ensure maximum quality and potency. They should not have any dead or decaying substances on them, as this is an indication that they are past their prime for use. Dried herbs will last longer than fresh ones; however, if you live in a dry climate, it is best to take precautions and put your herbs in a cooler location where they will not dry out due to lack of moisture in the air.

Tools Needed for the Making of Herbal Medicine

When choosing tools to use for the making of herbal medicines, there are a few things that need to be taken into consideration at the same time. These items include, but are not limited to the following:

You need to consider what type of herb you will be making, how many people will consume your herbal medicine, and how much time you have available.

When choosing tools, you will need to decide how many people will be consuming your herbal medicine. If it is for consumption by one person at a time, then a single piece of equipment should do all that it needs to. However, if you are taking medicine for a large group of people, then you will need to keep that in mind. If it is for more than one person at once, then you will need to look at having several pieces of equipment, which can each be used by the individual that needs them. Some examples of this would be containers that can hold herbs and tools that are used to make herbal medicines. Make sure to have plenty of containers on hand for any medicinal products that you will be making.

If time is an issue, then you will need to use the tool, which is the quickest for you to use. For example, if you work in the morning and must make your medicine before you leave, then a cheap tool that can be made in a short amount of time will be the best choice for you. However, if it is evening and you have time to spare before going home, then a more expensive tool may be better for you.

Making Herbal Medicine

When making herbal medicine during your leisure time, there are certain steps that should be taken to ensure that your herbal medicines are as effective as possible. These steps include, but are not limited to the following:

Choosing the amount of the herb to use, performing a cure-all on the herb, grinding up or chopping up your herbs, and finally, cooking and consuming.

When you are deciding how much of an herb to use, you should look at what kind of herbal medicine you would like to make. Some herbal medicine is meant to be consumed in a small dose, while others are meant to be consumed in large doses. However, each person's body is different, so some will need more medicine than others. This is determined by things such as age and overall health. As long as the herb is within the recommended dosage range, then it should be fine.

Once you have decided on how much of an herb to use, it is time to perform a cure-all that will help the herb become stronger and last longer. Depending on what herbal medicine you are making and what its intended use is, curing your herbs can be as simple as adding a few drops of herbal oil or tincture into it. However, there are more complicated cures that can be performed. These include extracting the properties from other plant materials or using animal products such as honey or milk to help with flavoring it.

Domestic herbalists choose a variety of herb plants and flowers found in their area to provide medicinal remedies for the common ailments that they experience.

1. Herbalists will observe which plants are the most common in their area and which are also known to grow near them. They will then use these homegrown or nearby herbs as opposed to purchasing those that are shipped from foreign countries.
2. To create medicine, an herbalist will use roots, stems, leaves, or fruit of fewer than ten or so plants at one time. This allows them to maintain biodiversity and better observe how these herbs react with each other.
3. Herbalists will prepare medicines along with the primary ingredients they use. For instance, if they use flowers, they will add a base such as honey, sugar, or vinegar so that the plant does not wilt.
4. Herbalists also add vitamin C to almost all of their medications. This vitamin helps preserve the color and prolongs a drug's effectiveness.
5. If the herb is poisonous, herbalists will only take a small amount of the liquid or powder they intend to use for treatment. This helps ensure that people do not get ill accidentally from consuming too much plant material.

What Is a Set?

A set is a group of medicinal plants bundled together that are meant to be used for one ailment. For instance, there may be a set of herbs meant to ease arthritis pain. If the herbalist feels that their arthritis medicine is not working as well as they had hoped, they may try another herbal set instead.

Why do some sets have more ingredients than others? On average, each herbalist will purchase about 30 to 40 sets per year. They will use each set only once or twice, so they have to be able to quickly determine what works and what does not before the plant wilts away.

How are sets organized? Herbalists group sets by their condition. For example, there might be a set for digestive problems, another for fevers, and another for headaches. But within these categories are usually a select few medicinal plants that herbalists believe do the most work for that ailment. Sets generally contain one or two plants from this foremost group of about ten herbs. This allows for more variation in treatment but also ensures that the herbalist is purchasing a good number of ingredients at once.

How many sets do domestic herbalists use? Herbalists usually purchase a selection of three to seven sets per year. This means that they will use about twelve sets per decade.

Sacred Medicine

What is sacred medicine? The term "sacred medicine" can be used to describe a variety of different methods, but in general, it refers to plants or other substances that are used for healing. In this sense, the concept of sacred medicine is similar to the idea of "natural remedies." Plants and other natural elements have been part of human life since our origins and have played a major role in tribal ceremonies and rituals. These are all subsets of what may be called "sacred medicine."

In the modern world, sacred medicine has become more diverse and widespread. The Ancient Greek historian Herodotus (484–425 BC) was one of the first to document the use of certain substances that we now recognize as sacred medicines. In his writings, he wrote about how to use various plants as remedies for various conditions. It was in this way that the use of many medicinal plants came to be regarded with religious significance.

Although it is difficult to pinpoint where these references occurred, they clearly exist in other ancient cultures as well. For example, the Ancient Egyptians used sacred medicine extensively. The use of sacred medicine in ancient Egypt was such that a person could be called a "physician," based solely on their knowledge of plants and their use as medicines.

Herbal doctors throughout the world have used many different plants for various purposes, some for healing and others for magic or divination. It is only recently, however, that modern westerners have begun to recognize the value of sacred medicine, and many experts are now working to preserve its diverse traditions. In addition to recognizing its importance in society and history, some modern medicinal professionals have begun to incorporate elements of sacred medicine into their practices.

Four Sacred Medicines in Indigenous Culture

There are four sacred medicines in an indigenous culture known as the Four Noble Ones. These medicines come from a plant, animal, mineral, or weather, and they have a powerful ability to heal.

These four medicines were first mentioned in Chinese literature about 2,200 years ago by the Taoist priest Chang Chung-Yuan. Much of what we know of them today comes from this Taoist tradition, but other cultures also speak of such a group of healing substances, including Daoists, Buddhists, and Islamic Muslims.

The four sacred medicines of the Four Noble Ones are:

The medicine of herbs (known as "dang shen" or "dang shen yin" in China, and also known as "yang shen" or "yang shen qi" in Taiwan.)

The medicine of the heavens (known as "tian sheng" or "tian xing" in China, and also known as "kai sheng" or "kai xing" in Taiwan.)

The medicine of animals (known by the Chinese name Qian Shen) is often translated into English as "bear's gallbladder," but it is not the same thing. "Qian" means "bear," and "Yin" means "gallbladder," but it does not mean "bear's gallbladder," but rather the medicinal properties of certain organs, such as gallbladder, liver, or kidney. In China is considered a medicine.

The medicine of minerals (known as "Sheng Ge") is often translated into English as "bone-marrow-fluid," but there is no such thing. This refers to an elixir made by extracting internal organs from animals and soaking them in resins to extract herbal oils. Traditionally, this was used for various ailments, including pneumonia. It is still used in Korea.

Traditional Chinese Medicine practitioners have used these four medicines for generations. Master Hu Hong-Yu is a well-known master of the "Wu Shu" (five animals) style of martial arts. He is also an herbalist (master of herbs or herbalism). He studied herbs with indigenous people in Taiwan until he was 22 years old and until he learned the knowledge of all the different herbs. Then he traveled to Buddhist temples and Taoist temples to learn their medical theories, their medical methods, and their medical language. At the age of 32, he began writing books about herbal medicine and traditional medical theory. Since that time, he has written more than twenty books.

The Taoist priest Chang Chung-Yuan, a Taoist priest from China, said that the human body is in balance if our internal fire is hot and our internal water is cold. If we can keep our internal fire hot and our internal water cold, then we are in perfect health. The four sacred medicines help us restore the balance of heat and cold in the body.

The medicine of herbs heals heat (yang) excesses (pores or holes of the skin are hot). This medicine penetrates deep into the body to stop inflammation and restore normal balance. It is also able to stop bleeding, stop pus, and help the body calm down.

The medicine of the heavens heals cold (yin) excesses (pores or holes of the skin are cold). This medicine is able to restore normal function and stop the pain. It can help stop excessive vomiting, diarrhea, and bleeding. This medicine also helps restore calm and stops excessive sweating.

The medicine of animals heals heat (yang) excesses (pores or holes of the skin are hot). It stops excessive sweating, restores normal function, and calms the body. This medicine also regenerates heat in general. It is used to relieve pain in joints, nerves, muscles, and tendons. It can reduce swelling. It is used to repair and prevent discharges in the blood, mucous membranes, and sinuses.

The medicine of minerals heals cold (yin) excesses (pores or holes of the skin are cold). It stops excessive bleeding, pain, and inflammation. What this medicine does is restore the normal function of the body. It draws out and eliminates toxins from the body. It also stimulates the flow of energy and the circulation of blood in the body. This medicine is used to protect the skin and prevent discharges in the nose, ears, and sinuses. It is used to repair and regenerate body parts, such as muscles, tendons, joints, nerves, and tendons.

The medicine of the heavens comes from heaven (Tai) and earth (sheng), according to the four seasons. It is a medicine that can cure many diseases by restoring the balance between yin (cold) and yang (heat). The herbs for this medicine come from heaven during spring, while the herbs come from the earth during summer. This is a medicine that must be gathered at three different times of the year. The herbs for this medicine come to us from the earth and are full of life. This medicine is given to patients who have a cataract or are suffering from a disease called "jaundice." This is very serious because it can make the patient blind.

The medicine of animals comes from heaven (Tai) and earth (sheng). It helps restore the balance between yang and yin in our bodies. Therefore, it cures many diseases by restoring the normal function of our body. The herbs for this medicine come to us from the earth during winter, while they come from heaven during summer. This is one of the most important medicines.

The medicine of minerals comes from heaven (Tai) and earth (sheng). It restores the normal function of the body. The herbs for this medicine come to us from the earth during winter, while they come from heaven during summer. This is a very important medicine because it can cure many diseases by restoring the normal function of our body.

These four medicines are used in Traditional Chinese Medicine because they are able to cause a change in disease by restoring the balance between yin and yang (heat and cold) as well as restore the flow of energy in our body due to the work these medicines do on our entire system. The herbs for these four medicines make up about 90% of traditional Chinese herbal medicine that is produced today.

Modern Sacred Medicine Movement

The modern sacred medicine movement is a diverse and healing movement that specializes in the spiritual benefits of traditional entheogenic substances.

These substances are used ceremoniously or ritualistically as a way to heighten awareness and see one more fully heal emotional wounds or connect with the world spiritually. Entheogens are considered sacraments by this church/movement because they provide direct spiritual experience when ingested correctly by those who tend to be seekers of religious experience and knowledge.

The modern sacred medicine movement is also a legal, political, and social movement that advocates for the use of these substances for healing and spiritual purposes. They are non-profit organizations that are part of the modern cannabis church movement as well as the free churches movement.

One method of cannabis administration in this branch is by smoking it at church services held by one of the many organizations in this field. The other methods include brewing it into teas or elixirs used as medicines or drinks for regular consumption—a common practice among some members of this branch is to consume marijuana tea each morning. Sublingual hash oil sprays have become popular among some members, especially those who suffer from cancers or HIV/AIDS. Some of these medical marijuana smokers that use sublingual sprays instead of smoking hash oil regularly come from a religious background. There are some churches and organizations that offer their services for free but must adhere to a tithe system in which the members of the church or organization pay dues to support the church or organization.

The modern sacred medicine movements conduct rituals and ceremonies wherever they gather, ranging from simple meetings at home to state-licensed university facilities.

The modern sacred medicine movement has been labeled "a fringe religion" by both the U.S. government and mainstream media outlets due to their stance on marijuana usage by patients suffering from certain illnesses while using it as a sacrament drug. As of today, most of the sacred medicine groups have not received mainstream media attention to a large extent because of the political and legal nature of the movement. Most mainstream religious publications either ignore this movement or only acknowledge it in passing. However, there are a number of people who have been able to obtain their medical marijuana cards after getting approval from their doctors for medical marijuana usage.

Along with cannabis use, some members prefer psychedelic mushrooms as a sacrament drug during their rituals and ceremonies. There are many churches that allow for members to partake along with cannabis or mushrooms on a daily basis while using these sacraments also in conjunction with topical medicines applied directly to the skin. These sacraments are used primarily for healing and spiritual purposes, but they can also serve as tools to ease the mental distress that can be associated with certain illnesses.

The main objective of this modern sacred medicine movement is to promote and educate people of all ages about the healing, recreational, and spiritual properties of cannabis. They believe that people should have the right to use these substances for medical purposes in accordance with their own beliefs and religious preferences. The modern sacred medicine movement promotes the legalization of these substances, as well as the decriminalization of marijuana in general.

Incorporating Native American Medicine in our Modern Lives

Introduction to New World Science

For most of us living in the 21st century, such a concept is out of reach. We depend on scientifically derived technologies to provide us with sustenance and shelter from nature's hostility. And yet, by using these same technologies, we have also created a world in which there are fewer and fewer places that have not been touched by human culture. This chapter makes it clear: Though this is the case, humanity could live in harmony with nature on Earth if we took special care to protect it against further degradation and damage.

The term "new world science" (NWS) has been used to describe science that is "contemporary," "different," and "innovative." Although NWS has been made with various meanings in mind, it is clear that the word has no specific meaning but rather points to a manner of thinking. New approaches and knowledge are being disclosed on a regular basis. In recent times, there have been numerous changes in science, technology, and the society that we live in. We must consider how to interpret them within our lifetimes and what action we should take to ensure their sustainability.

The Role of Native American Healing Traditions in Allopathic Medicine

In the early 1800s, John Ross established a medical school in Philadelphia. The American Medical Association (AMA) was founded in 1847 due to the need for better regulation of medicine. The AMA strictly adhered to allopathic philosophies, which held that "Western" medicine was superior to any other type of healing modality, including Native American healing traditions. Allopathic doctors have been quick to dismiss Native American healing traditions as superstition and primitive. Although they may not have had modern cultural practices, like acupuncture, many of these traditions still exist and are used regularly by people today for healing purposes.

According to the CDC, "In 2009, an estimated 1.9 million people had inter-tribal marriages" in the United States. Since there are more non-Native Americans marrying Native Americans, the numbers are increasing for people using alternative medicine, such as energy work, shamanism, and holistic healing practices taught by elders of native communities. There is a growing trend in America toward holistic health in general (no longer limited to just Native American populations) also. Traditions like sweat lodge ceremonies and sage hunting ceremonies are becoming more popular for people of all races and cultures to participate in as a means of reconnecting with nature and spirituality.

The Intersection of Traditional and Western Healing

Native herbal medicine, or indigenous healing, is a field that has been studied for centuries but only recently made its way to the mainstream. As the first force of traditional medicine from the earliest times up until the arrival of European settlers, it can be traced back to many ancient cultures, such as Aztecs and Native Americans. When Europeans arrived in America, white settlers began a systematic elimination and assimilation of native healers and natural medicines. Alcohol became an everyday part of many tribesmen's lives as they made a trade with nearby colonies for their deadly alcohol-based beverages at a rate that fueled both self-destruction and violence among them. In the past century, the emergence of western medicine has begun to dominate once again over indigenous practices. However, in recent decades, there has been a revival of interest in native healing practices, and many people have begun to appreciate them for their cultural value as well as their potential therapeutic benefits.

One key element of Native American medicine is that it is plant-based. Among many cultures in early America, plant knowledge was often passed down through generations by the mother or grandmothers because they were responsible for maintaining medicinal gardens and preparing herbal remedies for family illnesses.

There are more than 1,600 healing plants found throughout North and Central America, and many are still used today in traditional medicines (Rohrlich-Leavitt). This focus on holistic medicine is credited to the fact that Native Americans did not differentiate between the physical and the spiritual. They did not separate concepts of health and sickness from issues of harmony, balance, and spiritual beliefs (Fricke).

Many herbs used in indigenous healing were created by natural selection through trial-and-error over thousands of years. One example is "Lobelia inflate" or "Indian tobacco." The leaves can be smoked, chewed, steeped as a tea, or used in a poultice to treat gastrointestinal issues, including nausea and vomiting (Buhner). Tobacco is mildly toxic, but it was cultivated by many Native American tribes for centuries because. It also helps with indigestion, congestion, and other respiratory ailments.

Part III

~

Herbalism Encyclopedia & Apothecary I

Introduction

Native herbalism is a way of life that sets the foundation for many values and beliefs in the indigenous people of North America. It is not just about plants, but also about making sure all aspects of human life are taken care of. Native herbalists use a variety of plant materials to heal both physical and emotional ailments as well as promote spiritual growth.

A New Perspective about Native American Herbalism

In American culture, there are so many benefits associated with herbalism that it is easy to see how it has been used throughout history for medicinal purposes. There are several different ways that herbs have been used in North American culture, and there is a significant number of people who use herbs for medicinal purposes.

Herbs have been used to treat different types of illnesses. Some common ailments include headaches, colds, nausea, stomach cramps, bloating, and indigestion. It is also thought to be helpful if someone has a urinary tract infection or if they experience heartburn. They are also thought to be useful as natural remedies for skin issues such as psoriasis and eczema (Coalition for Ethical Medicine Web site). In addition to being used as a cure for illness, it is also thought that herbalism can help with emotional situations, such as stress or anxiety. Many herbalists believe that herbalism has the ability to help individuals get to know themselves better and in return, they can come closer to understanding their purpose in life.

Native American Herbalism is defined as "the use of plant materials to maintain health, prevent disease, or promote healing. In Native American culture, herbalism is a spiritual path practiced through the traditions of many tribes and peoples within Native America. It includes both traditional knowledge and practices relating to the healing properties of medicinal plants as well as a philosophy based on spirit and consciousness" (Smoking). The use of herbs for medicinal purposes appears to have been widely practiced by Native Americans since at least 7000 BCE. In the mid-1800s, tribes such as the Cherokee in North Carolina incorporated herbs used as a part of their traditional medicine (Greeley). The Navajo and Hopi Indians traditionally used cannabis as an herbal remedy to dull pain and aid in their hunting (Pourier).

The significance of herbs as a form of medicine played an important role in Native American culture. In the 1790s, the United States government began to study these indigenous remedies. However, it was not until 1897 that congress passed legislation designed to remove all federal restrictions on native medicines. This legislation marked the beginning of laws that allowed medicinal plants to be used by tribal members, doctors, and pharmacists without any restrictions.

There are many resources for exploring the practices of Native American herbalism, but few provide a comprehensive compilation of the knowledge. The Encyclopedia of Native American Herbalism in this manuscript is designed to fill that void. It is our hope that this resource will bring awareness and interest in the rich history and culture associated with these practices. This is not a cookbook or an instruction manual for use in treatment. Rather, it reflects a synthesis of information from ethnographic accounts, interviews with elders, personal experiences with plants such as peyote, and published botanical descriptions to create an understanding of how these plants are used by indigenous people in North America. This resource is designed to foster a deeper appreciation of the practices and knowledge associated with Native American herbalism.

Encyclopedia of Herbs

Medicinal native plants have been cultivated from the forest and have been introduced for decades to home gardens. The production and usage of such medicinal plants in modern times reflect a safer form of life for the homesteader community, as well as a safe re-supply strategy for the preppers and bug-out enthusiasts. Although these home remedies are never meant to take the place of qualified medical treatment, it's good to know that you're not powerless if you wind up by yourself. Below is a collection of 14 fantastic plants you'll find in the wild. Others can also be picked up at garden centers and attached to your own private garden for medication.

Parsley ("Petroselinum Crispum")

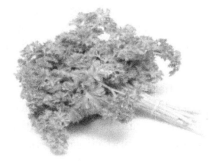

Parsley is a bitter, mild herb, which may boost your food flavor. Some find parsley to be just a curly green food garnish, but it really lets foods like stews produce a more natural taste. Parsley can help indigestion as an added benefit. Parsley is mostly grown annually, but it will stay evergreen all winter long in milder climates. Peregrine plants must mature to be large and bushy.

Parsley is an excellent source of vitamins A and C.

Mint ("Mentha")

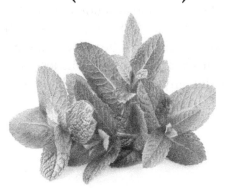

Mint types are numerous. It can be found in cocktails such as mojitos or mint juleps. Perhaps you can apply some mint to your iced tea for the season. Salt can freshen the air and help the stomach relax. But if you cultivate mint, note it's known as an unwanted herb. Mint spills over the greenhouse and takes over.

This is properly contained in barrels.

Dill ("Anethum graveolens")

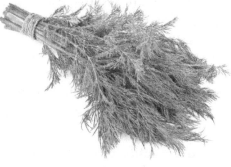

Dill is a great flavoring for fish, lamb, potatoes, and peas. It also assists in appetite and in preventing poor breath. It also has the additional benefits of minimizing swelling and cramps. It's easy to grow dill. It will draw helpful insects like wasps and other aggressive insects to your yard, too. It also saves a trip to Santa Barbara Dentist!

Thyme ("Thymus vulgaris")

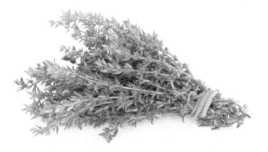

Thyme is a delicate herb in appearance. It is also used for potato, bean, and vegetable flavoring dishes. Thyme is widely found in cuisines like the Oriental, Italian, and Provençal countries. Combine it with potatoes, poultry, and lamb. Soups and stews are also flavored with thyme. It is a member of the family of mint. The most popular form is garden thyme with grey-green leaves and a minty, somewhat lemony scent.

Fennel ("Foeniculum vulgare")

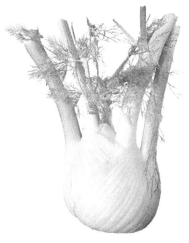

Fennel is highly flavorful and spicy, and it is the main component of absinthe and anise. Fennel is found in the Mediterranean region and grows well in dry areas near the coast or on the banks of the canal. The fennel's strongly aromatized leaves are similar in shape to dill. The bulb may be grilled, sautéed, or eaten raw. Fennel bulbs are used for garnishing or occasionally added to salads.

French Tarragon ("Fines herbes")

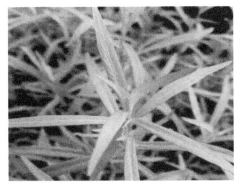

The main component of "Fines herbes" is the fresh tarragon, which is the aristocrat of fresh herbs. A must-have for every greenhouse with culinary herbs! It will transform an ordinary dish with its spicy anise flavor into a work of art. A little tarragon in a chicken salad creates a huge difference. The sauces, soups, and meat dishes are wonderful. Try on vegetables. Any hearty dish is the alternative.

Catnip ("Nepeta cataria")

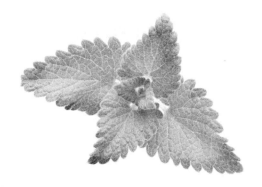

What's more enjoyable than seeing the family cat go somewhat berserk at the catnip smell? However, catnip is more than merely a stimulant to felines. It may be used both as a relaxant and a diuretic and laxative. When you buy catnip outside, mind that your cats love to crawl in and chew on it. Yet, having catnips in your backyard can be a disincentive to rodents, too.

Chives ("Allium schoenoprasum")

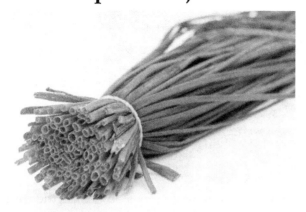

Chives belong to the family of garlic, which can be the best compliment to sour cream. Chives are often used for flavoring and are known to be one of French cuisine's "great herbs." Chives emerged in Asia but were used for about 5,000 years as an ingredient to add to milk. Eggs, fish, potatoes, salads, shellfish, and soups work well with chives. Chives are a healthy source of both beta-carotene and vitamin C.

Bay Leaves ("Laurus nobilis")

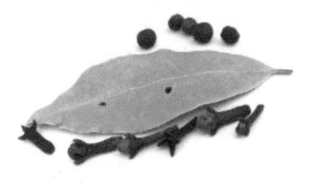

The fragrance of the noble leaves of the bay reminds you of balsam, clove, mint, and some even say, honey! Best known for its use in heart-rending stews and other long-simmering dishes with a very salty, peppery, and almost bitter flavor. At the start of the cooking process, add the whole leaves, and remember to remove them before serving. The sweet bay is of Mediterranean origin.

St. John's Wort ("Hypericum perforatum")

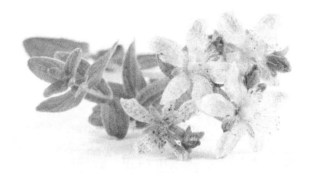

St. John's wort is thought to alleviate depression and anxiety symptoms, but it should not be considered a cure. It can help relieve muscle discomfort, too.

The term "wort" is an Old English word for "rose." The rose was called this as the flowers grow around the 24th of June, which is John the Baptist's birthday. St.

John's wort is also known as the weed; rosin rose, goatweed, chase-devil, or Klamath weed of Tipton. It is a common groundcover in gardens, as it is resistant to drought. This is a well-known herbal remedy for depression but not used in cooking.

Winter Savory ("Satureja montana")

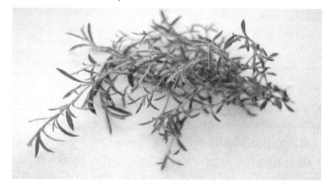

Winter savory, a deliciously sweet culinary spice, brings an enticing taste to several dishes. Its antibacterial and anti-fungal properties are also used medicinally. Winter savory, like its summer equivalent, is an aromatic mint family culinary herb that supplements the strong flavor of seafood, beans, and poultry. During the cooking process, while it loses some of this strength, winter savory retains aromatic qualities and is also used to spice liqueurs, creating a beautiful garnish to any salad.

Peppermint ("Mentha piperita")

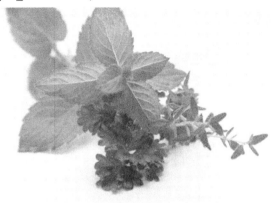

Like other mints, peppermint is popular for digestive help and air freshening.

Yet peppermint is also a healthy source of magnesium, potassium, and vitamin B. It is a combination mint and is a mix between water mint and spearmint. Peppermint oil may be used to spice but is effective as a natural pesticide as well. The symptoms of irritable bowel syndrome have been reported to decrease. Peppermint enjoys ample soil and part shade. It spreads easily like other mints, so try planting it in containers.

Stevia ("Stevia rebaudiana")

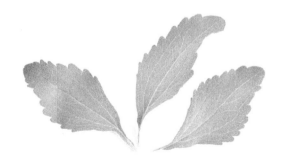

Stevia is an enticing plant in nature and a natural sweetener. The added benefit is that calories don't exist. Stevia is part of the sunflower family, which is native to the Western hemisphere's subtropical and tropical areas. Though it is a perennial plant, it can only thrive in North America's milder climates.

You can add stevia to your summer garden, anyway. Often known as "sweet leaf" or "sugar leaf," it is grown for its sweet berries. Stevia could

be used as a sweetener and as a replacement for sugar.

Lemongrass ("Cymbopogon")

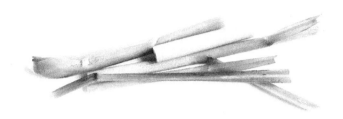

Lemongrass stalks can include antioxidants, such as beta-carotene, and protection against inflammation of cancer and eyes. Lemongrass has a good citrus flavor. You should brew it in tea and then use it as a spice for herbs. You need to stay in at least Zone 9 to expand the outdoors. Outside, it will grow up to 6 feet high, but if you grow it indoors, it would be significantly smaller.

Bergamot ("Bee Balm")

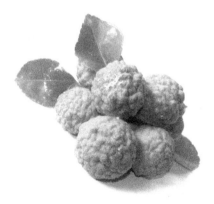

Bee balm is gaining revived popularity as a culinary plant, making it a perfect addition to pizzas, salads, bread, and other recipes that are complemented by the special taste of the plant. Bergamot is minty yet mildly sweet, rendering oregano a perfect alternative. Bergamot has a long tradition of being used by many Native Americans as a healing herb, including the Blackfeet. To treat small injuries and bruises, the Blackfeet Indians used this hardy herb in poultices. A tea manufactured from the plant has also been used to treat infections of the mouth and throat triggered by gingivitis, as the plant produces large amounts of a naturally occurring antiseptic (thymol) used in many brand name types of mouthwash.

Oregano ("Origanum vulgare")

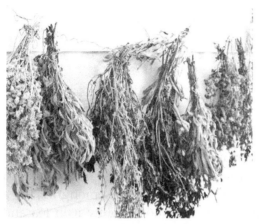

Oregano also belongs to the mint family and is native to Eurasia and the Mediterranean warm climates. Oregano is a seasonal herb that may be cultivated as an annual in colder climates. This is often referred to as wild marjoram and is loosely related to honey marjoram. Oregano is a favorite herb in Italian American food and is used for flavoring. It gained attention in the United States during World War II as troops came home with a taste for the "pizza herb."

Comfrey ("Symphytum")

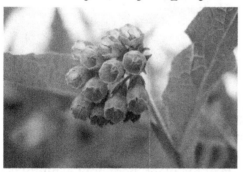

Cooked, mashed comfrey roots used as a topical remedy are good for inflammation, fractures, burns, and sprains. However, don't eat it; a new study suggests that eating in abundance is toxic to the liver. Root formulations are dangerous for internal usage owing to differences in the pyrrolizidine alkaloid content because they are considered pyrrolizidine-free. While the comfrey root is historically used for tea, the danger of its pyrrolizidine alkaloids is substantial. Therefore,

arrangements for comfrey root and young leaf need not be made in-house.

Burdock ("Arctium")

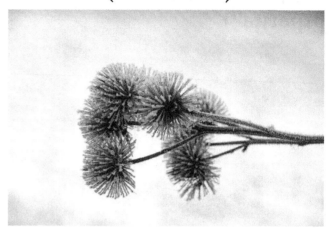

The roots and leaves form an outstanding tonic for the liver and help purify the body and blood. Most people use burdock root to help them get rid of acne symptoms, and that has a really good impact on a variety of skin issues, such as eczema. Render the dried root tincture in alcohol and drink 10–20 drops of tincture a day. Upon boiling them in water and discarding the water to eliminate bitterness, you may also consume the fresh leaves and roots.

Dandelion ("Taraxacum")

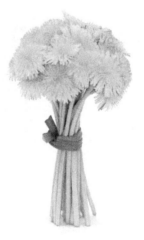

Place 1 teaspoon of the dried root in one cup of hot water as a general liver/gall bladder tonic and to promote digestion. A root-made tincture can be used three times a day. Some experts suggest tinctures dependent on alcohol since the bitter values of alcohol are more soluble. 1 or 2 teaspoons of dried leaves may be applied as a moderate diuretic or appetite stimulant to one cup of boiling

44

water and consumed as a decoction, up to 3 times a day.

Willow ("Salix babylonica")

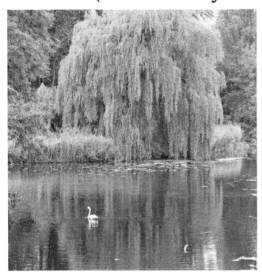

Use one which you can quickly recognize to prepare willow as a medicine.

Weeping willow grows in all of North America. Though not local, it thrives in any moist environment, and its droopy twigs and branches can be recognized. Over millennia, the leaves and the bark were used as medicine. To produce an astringent, boil a palm with green leaves in one cup with water for 10 minutes. If no other medicinal care is appropriate, soak a clean cloth in this brew and apply it directly to burns, abscesses, carbuncles, and ulcers.

Boil the bark scrapings off many twigs and boil them for 10 minutes in one cup of hot water for a gritty anti-diarrhea cocktail. Take a couple of sips every 2 hours, and then start until the effects go down.

The bark of many other willow family types, including the black willow, has been in use since 400 B.C. for inflammation and pain management.

Black willow bark, a precursor of aspirin, produces salicin. It was once normal for people to chew the pain and fever relief directly on the rasped bark.

Aloe Vera

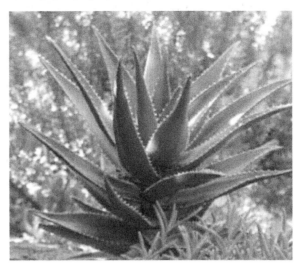

Common Name: Aloe

Botanic Name: Aloe vera L. (Aloe barbadensis Miller.)

Family: Asphodelaceae

Origin: South Africa and Arabian Peninsula

Other Names: Aloe from Barbados (Aloe vera). Aloe of the head (Aloe ferox)

Description

Aloe vera, Aloe barbadensis Miller (Aloe Vera L.), is a plant belonging to the genus Aloe and the Aloaceae family, modern and more specific classification introduced by Dr. Reynolds, instead of The previous wider subdivision of Liliaceae. It is a perennial plant belonging to the Xerophilous, called by the Arabs Alloeh, by the Chinese Alo-hei, took the name Barbadensis from Barbados Islands, despite its origin was the east coast of Africa. Today it is also found along the coasts of the Mediterranean. From its leaves is extracted a gel with multiple properties, which only since 1970 has been able to stabilize, preserving its effectiveness, thus helping to facilitate its spread. From Aloe leaves we extract a gel whose healthy properties and uses have been known since ancient times, even going back to the ancient Egyptians the first document that mentions its use: the "Egyptian book of remedies" of the famous Ebers papyrus (15th century BC). Cleopatra used Aloe gel for its properties for the beauty of the skin.

Properties and Indications

The drug is made from leaves. The outermost part of the leaves contains aloin, which has distinct laxative, purgative or tonic-digestive properties, depending on the dosage; the inner part contains a mucilaginous gel which is made up of 98.5% water, the remaining active substances.

The properties and uses of Aloe gel are very ancient, for its moisturizing, emollient, protective properties, able to maintain or restore the elasticity of the skin.

Aloe gel is an excellent cicatrizant; it has a draining and purifying function, as well as antiseptic and bacteriostatic. It also has anti-inflammatory properties. Its characteristics make it an excellent remedy against gastritis, ulcers, colitis; useful in case of rheumatism, acne, allergic reactions with special skin localization. For external use it is useful for dry and irritated skin, for mild burns and sunburn, to soothe razor fire, insect bites. The recommended use is both indoor and outdoor. Aloe vera juice without aloin can also be used during pregnancy and breastfeeding.

Achillea

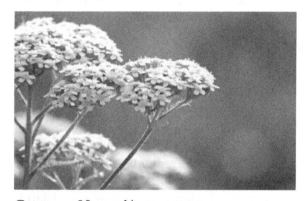

Common Name: Yarrow

Botanic Name: *Achillea millefolium L.*

Family: Asteraceae

Origin: Originally from Euphrasia, spread throughout Europe, America and Asia.

Other Names: EN: Yarrow

ES: Milenrama

FR: Millefeuille

DE: Gemeine Schafgarbe

Description

The drug consists of the flowering tops of Achillea M. millefolium L. (fam. Compositae), perennial herbaceous plant, rhizomatous, 30 to 50 centimeters high. It is cosmopolitan: it grows from the plain to the mountain areas, where it is commonly found in wet meadows, along ditches and hedges and in uncultivated places.

The flowering tops are harvested from June to September, they dry in the shade below 40 degrees, after gathering the inflorescences in bunches; they are preserved in paper or canvas bags.

Properties and Indications

Yarrow has emmenagogue properties; hemostatic; bitter-eupeptic; spasmolytic. The indications are therefore Amenorrhea and dysmenorrhea; Metrorrhagia; Anorexia and Gastrointestinal Dyspepsia; spasms of the digestive and uterine tract; venous affections (varices, phlebitis, hemorrhoids).

Precautions for Use

Since Achillea belongs to the Asteraceae family, it can cause allergic dermatitis in people who are particularly sensitive or allergic to plants of this family.

With regard to possible interactions, attention must be paid to its activity on blood clotting, especially for people taking anticoagulant drugs, whose action it could alter. In case of use to facilitate menstruation, if absent for various reasons, the use of Yarrow does not jeopardize a possible pregnancy ignored.

The use of Yarrow is not recommended during pregnancy and breastfeeding, and in children: some of its components may have a neurotoxic action.

Alpha-Alpha

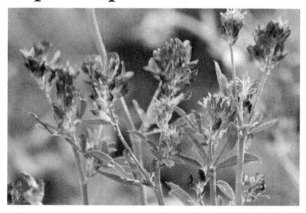

Common name: Alpha-alpha (pronunciation: Alpha-alpha)

Latin name: Medicago sativa L.

Other Names: Alfalfa, Spanish herb, Merica herb

Family: Belongs to the family of leguminous plants.

Description

Alfalfa, Medicago sativa, also called alfalfa, is a perennial herbaceous plant belonging to the family Leguminosae (or Fabaceae). It tolerates water imbalances well, as it develops roots up to 3-4 meters deep, giving rise to hollow stems up to one meter long, although the habit of mowing it regularly during the maximum

The vegetative period prevents normal growth. The leaves are trifoliate, but different from those of Clover (Trifolium pratense) because the central one has a petiole; the flowers gathered in the racemose inflorescence are blue-violet; the fruits are legumes containing from 2 to 6 very small seeds. The Alfalfa forms multi-annual forage meadows, called medicai, which produce numerous concentrated annual harvests during the flowering period.

The name Alfalfa derives from the Arabic al-fasfasa = forage plant, or from al-fal-fa = father of all foods. The genus name "Medicago" and the common name "medica," contrary to what can be assumed, do not allude to its use in medicine, but to the fact that the plant comes from the ancient Media, i.e. today's Iran.

Originally from South-West Asia, it also grows in the United States, especially in the Centre-North, where it is widely used as a forage plant, for the excellent nutritional properties that have earned it the name of "queen of forage plants," also because it prevents the meteorism of livestock. Like many leguminous plants, alfalfa is suitable for the green manure technique, to enrich the soil with nitrogenous substances, which are concentrated in their root tubercles.

Alfalfa today is used as food and/or as a natural energy supplement also by man, precisely because of its great nutritional properties, useful for the maintenance of well-being and health, as well as in cosmetics.

Properties and Indications

Alfalfa is rich in vitamin A, carotenoids, numerous B vitamins, including B12, as well as vitamins C, D, E, K, and PP; among the mineral salts include calcium, phosphorus, magnesium, potassium, iron, selenium, zinc, particularly present in its sprouts (seeds not sprouted should not be consumed), which are an excellent way to eat Alfalfa, in which the protein content is also high, about 30%, with a complete profile of all essential amino acids; Alfalfa also contains chlorophyll, saponins, phytoestrogens, and numerous digestive enzymes that promote assimilation.

Alfalfa leaf extract, rich in substances of very high biological value and of particular nutritional value, has tonic-energetic and phytonutrient properties, useful as a reconstituent in case of organic deterioration, malnutrition, weakness, convalescence, asthenia and lack of appetite, thanks to its remineralizing and reconstitutive action due to its high nutritional power. It can also be indicated in menopause for the presence in its composition of isoflavones and cumestrol, a substance that exerts a phytoestrogenic activity that shows a great affinity for the cellular receptor of estrogen.

For the antioxidant action carried out by bioflavonoids, flavones, vitamins C, E, K, PP, and for the content in chlorophyll, Alfalfa protects the skin and connective tissues, strengthens fragile capillaries, counteracts anemia. The content of saponins, able to bind to cholesterol, helps to decrease LDL cholesterol levels and fight atherosclerosis, while the presence of the alkaloids asparagine and trigonelline helps to modulate blood glucose levels.

Alfalfa has been known for two thousand years by the ancient Chinese and Persian medicine, and by the Indian Ayurveda that recommends it to promote digestion and as an antimeteoric, as an anti-inflammatory to relieve arthritis and to increase lactation in the nurse. Its natural fluorides, anti-cariogenic, fight caries and strengthen teeth.

Alfalfa is recommended as a dietary supplement to provide energy in case of intense physical activity, to supplement vegetarian and vegan diets, as a detoxifier, anti-anemic, ant cholesterol and hypoglycemic, to combat digestive disorders. In cosmetics we use seed extract, which contains a phytocomplex rich in saponosides, with regenerating and redensifying activity on the skin; it also contains phytostimulins, Bio catalyzing substances with healing and antioxidant properties.

Alfalfa extract is used in phytocosmetics for the preparation of anti-wrinkle creams and serums, and as an elasticizer, toning and firming to prevent stretch marks.

Precautions for Use

Alfalfa supplements are contraindicated in the presence of gout, if you take antidiabetic drugs, synthetic hormone therapies, and also in conjunction with anticoagulant drugs, for the presence of vitamin K that could reduce the effect.

Devil's Claw

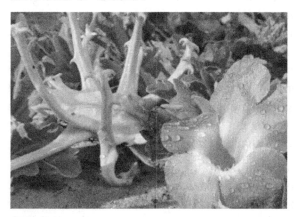

Description

The drug is the secondary root of Harpagophytum procumbens (Burch) DC. (Fam. Pedaliaceae), an herbaceous plant that grows wild in the Kalahari Desert. The name of the genus comes from the Greek "Harpago" (=rampino) and alludes to the fruits provided with hooks that attach themselves to the legs of the animals, thus spreading the seeds. The root of the plant is formed by a taproot, called primary root, which penetrates vertically into the ground, and secondary roots that are dispersed for a radius of about 1.5 meters around the plant.

Properties and Indications

The Devil's Claw is anti-inflammatory, analgesic, anti-rheumatic.

It is therefore indicated in cases of chronic rheumatism, rheumatoid arthritis, osteoarthritis with different localization (coxarthrosis, gonarthrosis, and cervical arthrosis), joint pain in general, tendinitis, and neuritis on a traumatic basis. The analgesic and anti-inflammatory properties of the plant have been widely confirmed by recent studies.

The activity of the drug is often referred to its main compound, the harpagoside; however, as with most drugs, the administration of the single active ingredient does not exactly reproduce the activity observed with the phytocomplex "in its entirety."

Precautions for Use

For its bitter-tonic action, it is advisable to take the Devil's Claw on a full stomach, if you have inflammation of the stomach mucosa and, like all bitters, should be avoided in case of ulcer. The use is also discouraged in case of taking anticoagulant drugs and during pregnancy.

Bee Pollen

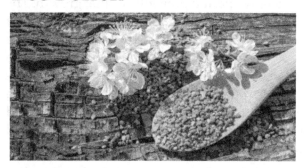

The pollen derives its name from the Latin pollen, or fior di farina. It is in fact presented as a powder of variable color (yellow-red). The pollen consists of microscopic structures to which plants entrust the transport of their germ cells. The bees collect it and use it for the production of royal jelly and for feeding the larvae. Bee pollen is the richest and most complete source of minerals, vitamins, enzymes and amino acids in nature. In fact, it contains:

- 21 of the 23 known amino acids.
- Minerals such as Potassium, Calcium, Magnesium.
- Proteins (35% of pollen content).
- Vitamins, especially A, B, C and E.
- Carotenoids, flavonoids and phytosterols.
- All essential trace elements.

10 Reasons to Take Pollen

1. It is a nutritional dynamo, a pure and immediately available source of energy.
2. It is anti-aging: it is rich in nucleic acids, essential for cell growth, repair and detoxification.
3. Improves the skin: pollen is used both for its rejuvenating effect and to treat skin problems such as acne and dehydration.

4. Helps to lose weight. Pollen reactivates lazy metabolism and suppresses appetite at the same time. In addition, the high Lecithin content helps to eliminate fat from the body.

5. Helps keep cholesterol under control thanks to the presence of phytosterols. Pollen lowers the so-called bad cholesterol, and raises the good cholesterol, decreasing the risk of stroke and heart disease.

6. Improves sports performance, allowing you to use energy more efficiently. Pollen increases strength, endurance, and recovery speed.

7. Being a stimulant, pollen also increases libido and sexual arousal.

8. It stimulates the brain, increasing concentration, mental lucidity and memory by up to 40%.

9. Strengthens the immune system, increasing the number of white blood cells, lymphocytes and gamma globulins in the blood. It also has antibiotic properties.

10. It is a support for anticancer therapies: it reduces the negative effects of radiation and chemotherapy, and increases the number of immune cells, to better fight tumors.

Bach Flowers

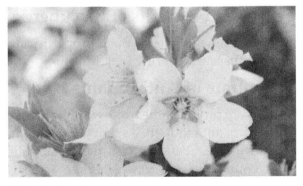

Description

Body health and mood are not split. Bach flowers work on both fronts and each of them is suitable for different personalities, produces effects and works on emotions in different ways. Let's see them one by one. Some people are predisposed to certain emotions rather than others. Some people tend to be hyperactive, while others let themselves go into inertia. Edward Bach indicated for each state of mind the most suitable floral remedy. Bach had understood that, for example, a person with the fear of losing control could never be treated and cured as someone who wanted to overcome a trauma of any nature. Healing through the flowers of Bach therefore also pushes us to know better who we are deep down, through that delicate phase that is the choice of the remedy that suits us.

Benefits and Contraindications

Bach flowers do not cure the disease but are aimed to unlock the reactive force of an individual and mobilize the inner forces to trigger a positive change. The essence indicated works on rebalancing negative emotional attitudes that promote the onset of various disorders. Taking care through the Bach flowers therefore also pushes us to know better who we are deep down, through that delicate phase that is the choice of the remedy that suits us. Bach flowers are particularly suitable for children because they do not give side effects, do not create addiction, you cannot go into hyper dosage. On the contrary, it can be said that children are the best users of Bach flowers because they have no preconceptions and react quickly and lastingly. There are no particular contraindications, except for what is called the crisis of awareness, consisting of an exacerbation of symptoms just before healing.

Bees Wax

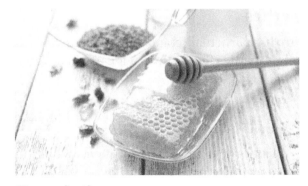

Description

Bee product par excellence, in addition to honey and propolis, beeswax is a secretion of the homonymous small insects (Apis mellifera), with which they build the internal structures of the hive (honeycomb) where the honey is stored. The use of beeswax dates back to the ancient Egyptians who used it in mummification processes and in the production of their ships, as it was widespread in the Roman populations who used it to protect their paintings from water and humidity.

For many years, therefore, beeswax has been a material of enormous importance for man, being the only available natural product of its kind. Nowadays, the field of application of beeswax has narrowed, as it has been replaced by similar, sometimes less expensive, materials.

However, this does not mean that beeswax has lost its value. In fact, beeswax is a by-product of honey extraction: it is believed that bees have to fly 530,000 km to collect a kilo of honey.

Types of Beeswax

According to the procedures to which it is subjected after its collection, we can distinguish two types of beeswax, whose uses are however superimposable:

- Yellow wax: it is the wax that is obtained by simple collection and extraction from the honeycomb. It is yellow in color and is characterized by its typical and pleasant aroma.

- Sunrise wax: it is obtained through the purification and bleaching of yellow wax through the action of air or through the action of chemical agents such as chlorine, chromic acid, hydrogen peroxide, etc. Normally, Alba wax does not have the delicate and pleasant aroma that characterizes untreated yellow wax.

Properties

Due to its particular composition, beeswax has several properties that allow a wide use in different sectors.

In detail, beeswax is equipped with:

- Emollient properties;
- Water-repellent and protective properties (since it forms a kind of film on the surface on which it is applied);
- Emulsifying properties.
- In antiquity, moreover, it was believed that beeswax also had healing properties and, for this reason, it was applied hot (and then melted) on wounds, in order to facilitate healing.

However, most likely, beeswax could facilitate the healing of wounds, not because it had real healing properties, but because it was able to create a barrier to protect the wound from the external environment while preventing the development of possible infections.

Blackberry

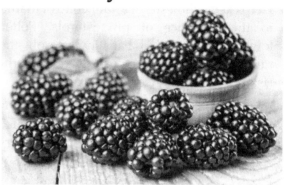

Description

Blackberry is the fruit of the bramble tree, whose scientific name is Rubus ulmifolius, a plant belonging to the large Rosaceae family which includes many other fruit plants such as apple, pear, almond, peach and apricot. It grows spontaneously in the countries of the Mediterranean basin. Walking along country roads it is very common to come across large thorny bushes that in summer fill up with these succulent berries. Today, blackberries are widely cultivated in Eastern Europe and the United States. The fruits are harvested between July and September depending on the variety. Summer is therefore the best season to enjoy them.

Properties and Benefits of Blackberries

Let's see in detail what are the main properties and benefits that these fruits bring to our health.

A Concentrate of Antioxidants

Blackberries are probably the fruits with the highest content of antioxidant agents, including anthocyanins, catechins, tannins, quercetin, gallic acid that counteract the action of free radicals, highly reactive molecules responsible for cellular processes underlying degenerative diseases. Tannins have anti-inflammatory and vasoconstrictive action, i.e., they narrow blood vessels by accelerating the healing of any wounds.

Good Source of Vitamins

They are rich in vitamin C, also a powerful antioxidant, which performs key functions in many fundamental physiological processes, including the immune response. They also contain vitamin A (involved in the processes of vision, cell differentiation and embryonic development), vitamin E which protects the skin and vitamin K, which is important for bone health and regulates blood clotting mechanisms. B vitamins are also well represented, including folic acid, so their consumption is recommended during pregnancy.

Rich in Fiber

Their particular conformation, in the form of aggregates of small round fruits, called drupes, makes blackberries particularly rich in fiber, both soluble and insoluble (100 g of blackberries contain 5.3 g of total fiber). Among the soluble fibers, we find pectin, which helps to reduce the levels of cholesterol in the blood and assists digestive processes, as well as promoting the absorption of glucose and therefore improves blood glucose levels. Insoluble fibers instead facilitate intestinal transit and give a sense of satiety.

Rich in Mineral Salts

Blackberries have a high copper content, an important mineral for the metabolism of bones and red and white blood cells. Magnesium, calcium, iron, zinc and manganese are also well represented.

Low-Calorie

With only 43 calories per 100 g, blackberries provide a full supply of energy with a low glycemic index and can therefore also be freely consumed by diabetics. Diuretics thanks to their good potassium and water content (88%), blackberries have moisturizing and purifying properties.

Blackberries: Suggestions for Use

Unfortunately, due to their easy perishability, it is difficult to find fresh blackberries on the market, but they can be easily purchased frozen. In summer we can find them by walking through the woods, probably the best places to pick them. After careful cleaning, we can eat them alone or add them to a yogurt or ice cream, or, if we have a good quantity, transform them into a jam or a jam that we can use to garnish our tarts even in winter. If you buy or collect them fresh you can keep them in the refrigerator for a couple of days at most, but a useful piece of advice is to eat them immediately.

Buckbrush

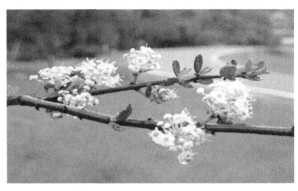

You need somewhere around one of your kidneys to work appropriately to live, and outstanding amongst other regular components to guarantee that your kidneys work well is the buckbrush.

Moreover, buckbrush can likewise be utilized to treat tumors and pimples, aggravation and sore throats.

The most ideal approach to burn-through it is to make tea from it. Essentially heat up some water and put the roots in for five to ten minutes. You would then be able to continue to drink the subsequent buckbrush tea to get the full advantages.

Black Raspberry

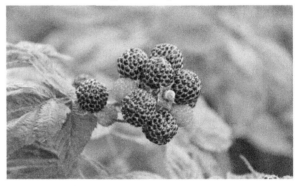

Description

The composition of black raspberries cannot be compared to the composition of red berries or blackberries. A lot of precious substances are included.

1. The high content of vitamin R in black raspberries helps to strengthen the walls of blood vessels.

2. Anthocyanins present in the fruit have strengthening effects of antisclerosis and capillary on the body. They can improve visual

acuity and skin condition by acting as powerful antioxidants.

3. The branches and leaves of the plant contain coumarins, which improve blood coagulability and reduce the amount of prothrombin in the body.

4. The high content of black raspberry protein that is able to ensure normal metabolic processes in the body and promote cell development and formation.

5. The combination of folic acid and vitamin C protects the body from harmful substances, oxidation in the body, slows down the aging process and strengthens the immune system. In addition, vitamin C contributes to better absorption of iron, which is contained in many raspberries. That is why the berry is so useful for blood diseases, especially anemia.

6. The high fiber content of black raspberries has a positive effect on the digestive tract, eliminating chronic or temporary constipation.

7. Pectins are substances that contribute to the elimination of harmful and toxic substances from the body, slag, heavy metals.

8. Organic acids rich in black raspberry, including citric, malic, ascorbic, are very important for the body. They effectively remove radionuclides.

9. Beta-sitosterol acts as an obstacle on the walls of blood vessels for the deposition of cholesterol. This component is a kind of prevention of sclerosis. The same substance can boast and plant leaves.

10. Salicylic acid or vitamin B9 has a bactericidal effect on the body.

11. The higher the maturity of the berries, the more salicylic acid they contain.

12. Magnesium in large amounts improves cardiac function.

The berries contain about 12% sugar, 3% are organic acids, their salts, coloring substances and tannins, up to 0.9% is occupied by pectins, 4-6% is given to cellulose, there are B vitamins and PP, ascorbic acid and folic acid up to 45 mg are also included iodine, essential oil, fatty acids, carotene and other substances.

The composition also includes:

- Macro-microelements: manganese, copper, iron, phosphorus, zinc.
- Vitamins A, groups B, E, PP.

Useful Properties of Black Raspberry for Human Body

Despite their rarity, black raspberries are still used as medicine for home treatment. The abundance of valuable berry qualities is due to its chemical composition.

1. Black raspberry is used as an antipyretic agent. It can be used to treat ARVI, sore throat and colds.

2. You should use raspberry berries to clean the blood and improve its condition.

3. Raspberry drugs are considered anti-inflammatory, analgesic, antiemetic, antitoxic and hemostatic.

4. Black raspberry has a beneficial effect on the organs of the digestive system. Berry is able to cure diseases and relieve stomach pains, eliminate intestinal problems and improve appetite.

5. Blackberry is suitable for the treatment of beriberi and strengthens the entire immune system as a whole. To do this, it is best to eat berries in spring to protect yourself from viral infections, colds and saturate your body with vitamins.

6. Berries are useful for the cardiovascular system.

7. Raspberry is used in the treatment of home bladder, the berry relieves swelling.

8. A decoction of berries can reduce inflammation of the oral cavity and treat sore throat.

9. The berry is used in the treatment of gynecological diseases and infertility.

10. Black raspberries are appropriate for the treatment of diabetes.

11. With hypertension, it helps the regular consumption of juicy berries. They do not provide a one-time effect, but lasting and long-lasting results.

12. In all kinds of medicine, black raspberry is recognized as the best medicine that can treat

respiratory diseases, relieves colds and inflammation, cough and runny nose.

13. Black Raspberry is a prophylactic agent for cancer. An antioxidant agent has an antitumor effect on the body.

14. Black raspberry tea will help normalize the menstrual cycle in women and reduce pain during this period.

15. Berry is actively used in cosmetology as an ingredient for facial masks. Raspberries mixed with yogurt or sour cream will relieve skin with fine wrinkles and improve its condition.

Black Raspberry: Useful Properties

Well, here I ask who does not know raspberries. Everybody knows it! Red fragrant berries from forests and gardens, firmly established on our table in the form of jam, compotes and jelly. Its place in folklore, from folk tales to mischievous songs, has always been associated with beauty, sweetness and delicate taste.

What if, for example, you ask about the beneficial properties of raspberry black? The answer will be simple—this is not a raspberry, but a blackberry! And this is wrong!

Black raspberry exists and despite its similarity to blackberry, it is a separate type of raspberry. Native of black raspberry from North America. It came to us recently and can only be reached by some of the most advanced amateur gardeners. At the same time, they know it well in Europe. The most popular black raspberries received in the UK, especially in Wales, France and Poland. It is also found among Japanese gardeners.

Buckwheat

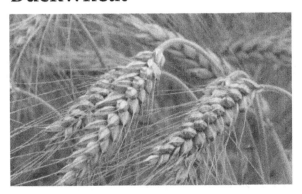

Description

Buckwheat or "black wheat" (Polygonum fagopyrum) is a flowering plant that does not belong to the Gramineae family but to the Polygonaceae family. However, it is commercially placed among cereals, because it has strong similarities with the species belonging to this group, both for the qualitative and technological characteristics of the grain (nutritional content and food use) and for the cultivation techniques. However, it is considered a minor cereal and belongs to that group of crops that have suffered, over the years, an increasingly reduced spread due to several factors, first of all, the lower productivity compared to wheat but also a standardization of consumption and therefore a lower demand on the market.

Largely cultivated in the past, its cultivation has been progressively abandoned, so much so that the flour currently on the market is obtained from the milling of wheat imported from China. Recently, however, there has been a reversal of the trend: minor cereals are crops that offer the possibility of limiting production costs or are characterized by a limited demand for technical means and also allow you to exploit the marginal areas of our territory, difficult to cultivate. Buckwheat is a wild plant that grows in the areas of Siberia and Manchuria and was introduced in the West during the Middle Ages. According to the first theory, the Turks introduced the plant in Greece and the Balkan Peninsula and from this, the name buckwheat, i.e., wheat of the Turks or Saracens, is derived.

The second theory claims that the spread occurred through Asia and Northern Europe because of the migrations of Mongolian peoples who, from southern Russia, brought the wheat to Poland and Germany, from where it would spread to the rest of Europe. It is likely that both theories are valid and that the propagation took place simultaneously from both North and South. Today it is still widespread in Russia, while in Europe it is limited to parts of France and Germany. In the production of flour, triangular grains can be ground keeping the cuticle. The flour that is obtained from milling is also called "bigia" because of its characteristic dark-grey color. If, on the other hand, the grains are used whole, for soups or cold salads, they must be peeled, i.e., freed from the black cuticle. The whole plants are also used by farmers as fodder or litter for livestock. In addition, bees get dark and very tasty honey from buckwheat flowers.

Properties and Benefits

Buckwheat is very important for its nutritional characteristics. It differs from common cereals by the high biological value of its proteins (14.1% compared to 9.2% of common wheat and 8.5% of corn flour) which contain the eight essential amino acids in optimal proportions, while "real cereals" contain little lysine. Lysine, an essential amino acid, is present in high percentages, higher than those of egg and all other cereals, with values varying between 4 and 20% depending on the cultivars and environmental conditions.

Compared to wheat flour, buckwheat flour is gluten-free and is therefore suitable for foods for celiacs. Buckwheat is a good source of fiber and minerals, it is very rich in phosphorus, calcium (more than wheat), iron, copper, magnesium, manganese and its percentage of potassium exceeds that of all other cereals, it also contains important vitamins such as those of group B (B1, B2, PP, B5).

Cayenne

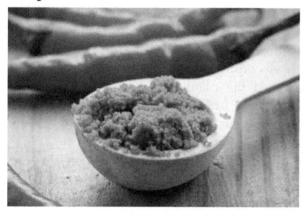

Cayenne pepper is considered one of the main foods of the Hunzas in Asia (along with apricots and millet), this wonderful spice, taken regularly, acts as an immune stimulant and anti-inflammatory.

15 Benefits of Cayenne Pepper

In addition to the power to relieve discomforts such as toothache and seasickness and alleviate the symptoms of fever, malaria and alcohol addiction, it reduces the pain caused by Herpes, osteoarthritis, rheumatoid arthritis. It is also considered a valuable aid against lazy bowel and stomach pain,

so it is an excellent natural remedy for cramps and diarrhea. Let's go hours to learn more about all its properties through a more detailed list:

Fights Colds and Flu

Cayenne pepper is a natural source of beta carotene and antioxidants that support your immune system. It helps to disintegrate and remove congested mucus and once it has left the body, flu and cold symptoms decrease. In addition to helping you fight flu symptoms, cayenne pepper increases your body temperature, which makes you sweat and thus stimulates the activity of your immune system.

Acts Positively Against Allergies

As recently referenced, cayenne pepper is a calming specialist, ready to forestall hypersensitivities and manifestations identified with them. A food hypersensitivity, for instance, is a quantifiable reaction to the utilization of a specific food. Food hypersensitivities or prejudices can be brought about by an illness called intestinal penetrability, which permits proteins and food particles to go through the intestinal dividers causing fundamental irritation of the body.

It Relieves the Pain Caused by Migraines

The fruit of the chili plant contains a chemical agent called capsaicin. Capsaicin has been studied to assess whether its ability to reduce the feeling of pain was effective. Researchers suggest that cayenne pepper, thanks to its hotness, is able to stimulate a response to pain in a different part of the body. When this happens, the brain focuses its attention on that new point and stops focusing on the head pain that causes migraines.

After this initial reaction, the nerve fibers exhaust substance P or pain substance, and the sensation is reduced. Basically, it is deceiving the body, making him believe that he feels discomfort elsewhere so that the head is no longer the focus of the pain chemists.

Source of Vitamin A and Vitamin E

Vitamin A and vitamin E are natural antioxidants that play a critical role in maintaining visual health, neurological function and healthy skin, reducing inflammation and fighting free radicals.

Fortunately for us, cayenne pepper is a great resource of both vitamins.

Helps Digestion

One of the greatest benefits of cayenne pepper is its positive effect on the digestive system. It stimulates both the production of saliva, stimulating the salivary glands necessary for the activation of the digestive process and the production flow of enzymes essential for proper functionality. So it is important both for good digestion and to prevent bad breath. It also regulates the production of gastric juices that support the body's ability to metabolize food and toxins.

Promotes the Health of the Cardiovascular System

Clots are blockages in your arteries and blood vessels that restrict blood flow through the circulatory system. Cayenne pepper encourages fibrinolytic activity and helps prevent clots. It is also the reason why it is effective in preventing heart attacks: the capsaicin in cayenne pepper helps to sweep away lipid deposits (which cause the arteries to narrow) so that they dilate along with the blood vessels, sweeping away clots.

Relieves Pain in Nerves and Joints

Studies have found that Cayenne relieves post-operative pain such as that of mastectomies and amputations. It also relieves pain resulting from nerve damage to the feet or legs due to diabetes, low back damage, as well as fibromyalgia symptoms such as joint and muscle pain.

Promotes Sweating

Another of the less considered effects is that the regular consumption of this chili develops an additional purifying capacity, able to promote drainage through sweat since there is a gradual increase in body temperature.

Possible Anticancer Agent

According to some studies, capsaicin may have its role as a natural remedy for cancer, including the treatment of prostate cancer.

Studies show that this important ingredient in cayenne pepper is able to inhibit the growth of cancer cells and prevent the activation of dangerous new formations.

Other studies show that cayenne pepper is effective in preventing lung cancer in smokers. The high level of capsaicin present in Cayenne may slow the formation of tobacco cancers. Similar effects have also been obtained in the study of liver cancer when exposed to it.

Useful for Slimming and Eliminating Excess Fat

As one of the key anti-inflammatory foods, the benefits of cayenne pepper also extend to the dietary area. Studies show that consuming cayenne pepper for breakfast generates less appetite so you are led to consume fewer calories during the day. It also burns excess fat because it is a metabolic stimulator. It improves metabolism in general and takes away the sense of hunger. Cayenne pepper also has abilities in regulating metabolism. In addition to suppressing the sense of hunger (a quality we just talked about in the previous paragraph) it regulates blood glucose levels, keeps blood pressure levels balanced and helps the body to lower LDL cholesterol and triglycerides.

It Has Antifungal Properties

Cayenne pepper has the ability to kill mushrooms and prevent the formation of pathogenic ones. Studied to determine in vitro its antifungal activity, it has given surprising results: it is active against 16 different strains of fungi including Candida.

Candida is a fungus that supports nutrient absorption and digestion when at appropriate levels in the body. When overproduced, however, the typical symptoms of Candida appear in the form of hormonal imbalance, joint pain, digestive problems and weakness of the immune system.

Natural Remedy Against Cellulite

Cayenne pepper is a thermogenic agent, able to increase the temperature of the body so as to promote the natural ability of the body to dispose of fat. This combined with other beneficial effects towards circulation makes cayenne pepper effective in facilitating the elimination of cellulite.

Preliminary Studies Also Show Benefits for Psoriasis

It is a chronic inflammatory skin disease. In sick subjects, the epithelial cells reproduce too quickly and the result is swollen areas under the skin covered with whitish scales at the top.

Two experiments show that 0.025% of a capsaicin-based cream (from cayenne pepper) for local use is effective in the treatment of psoriasis. The first study shows a significant decrease in scales and redness over a six-week period in 44 patients with moderate and severe forms of psoriasis. The second is a double-blind study of 197 patients. Psoriasis was treated 4 times a day for six weeks with capsaicin cream, with a significant decrease in scales, thickness, redness and itching.

Protects the Stomach

Cayenne pepper has excellent anti-irritant properties that make it effective in relieving ulcers, stomach pain and coughs. The common thought is that cayenne pepper, when consumed in excessive amounts, develops stomach ulcers due to its irritating and acid secretive nature. People with ulcers do indeed have an indication to avoid or at least limit its use; however, recent more research has revealed that capsaicin is not only the cause of the formation of ulcer symptoms but also something to rely on for treatment. In fact, it has been shown that cayenne pepper does not stimulate, but inhibits the secretion of acids, stimulating instead alkaline and mucus secretions and in particular the flow of gastric mucosa in the blood, which helps in the prevention and treatment of ulcers.

Easy to Integrate into Any Diet

The cayenne pepper is marketed in many ways, starting with the real chili, as a supplement or as a spice. It is precisely the versatility of this food that makes it extremely easy to use: as a salad dressing or to flavor your dishes. Those who love the spicy flavor will certainly not be disappointed.

Cattail

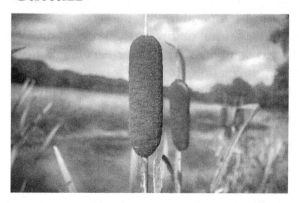

Cattail is even more a preventive treatment rather than a real medication.

All aspects of the plant can be eaten aside from the seeds and leaves.

Cattail is best utilized as a cleaner for fresh injuries like cuts, scraped areas and scratches. Essentially open the base of the cattail and carry it into direct contact with the serious injury, then, at that point secure it with a string or paracord.

What's more, cattail debris can be utilized for this equivalent restorative reason.

Essentially carry it into direct contact with the fresh injury.

Chamomile

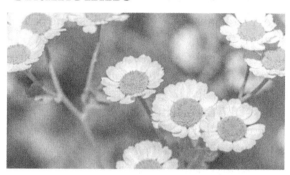

Description

An aromatic plant with bushy habit generally does not exceed 50 cm in spontaneous forms, while in cultivated varieties it can reach 80 cm.

It has several stems starting from the base, more or less branched in the upper portion and a taproot. The leaves are alternate and sessile, oblong, with lamina is bipennatosette or tripennatosette, with very narrow linear laciniae. The flowers are grouped in heads with a conical and hollow receptacle, the outer ones have white ligula, and the inner ones are tubular with yellow corolla. The flower heads with a diameter of 1-2 cm are grouped in corymbose tops.

Properties of Chamomile

With chamomile flowers are prepared infusions notoriously used for their mildly sedative virtues. In fact, the plant has no hypnoinductive active ingredients, like most medicinal herbs used against insomnia, but on the contrary, it has mainly antispasmodic properties, such as lemon balm, i.e. it produces muscle relaxation, due to the presence in its phytocomplex of flavonoids (eupatuletin, quercimethrin) and coumarins. These combinations of active ingredients make chamomile an excellent myorelaxant, useful in case of intestinal cramps, poor digestion, irritable bowel syndrome, muscle spasms and menstrual pain, but also in case of nervous tension and stress because it causes a feeling of pleasant relaxation with a calming effect on nervousness and anxiety. The herbal teas obtained with this plant eliminate intestinal gases and promote digestion, producing a general improvement in the functions of the gastroenteric system.

Like mallow, chamomile has good natural anti-inflammatory properties, thanks to the protective action on the mucous membranes exerted by the mucilage and the components of its essential oil (azulene and alpha-bisabolol). For this reason, it is used as a soothing, decongestant, softening and calming remedy, in all types of irritations of external and internal tissues: dermatitis, wounds, ulcers, and gastritis, conjunctivitis, and rhinitis, irritations of the oral cavity, gingivitis and urogenital inflammation. The plant is also used successfully as a painkiller in case of toothache, sciatica, headache, back and cervical pain. This is thanks to organic acids (salicylic acid, oleic acid, stearic acid) and lactones, which give it antiphlogistic virtues similar to those of cortisone. Recent studies have also shown the hypoglycemic effects, useful to lower the level of sugar from the blood, as it inhibits the transformation of glucose into sorbitol, responsible, when in excess, for damage to the eyes, kidneys and nerve cells, which are found in people suffering from diabetes.

Contraindications

The intake and use of chamomile tea have no particular contraindications. The only side effects that may occur are related to possible allergic reactions due to the presence of sesquiterpene lactones in the plant.

Chokecherry

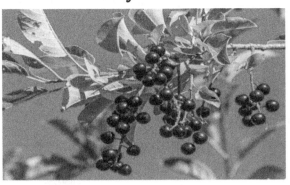

Description

Considered by Native American tribes as an all-purpose medical treatment, the berries were pitted, dried, and ground into a tea or poultice to treat a variety of ailments. These include coughs, colds, flu, nausea, inflammation and diarrhea. As an ointment or poultice, it is used to treat burns and wounds. The chokecherry pit—as much as apple seeds—are poisonous in high concentrations. Be sure to box the cherries if you are thinking of this for any use.

Chokecherry owes its activity mainly to the presence of the glycoside cyanidrinic prunasin and its cleavage products for which the drug has a depressing and calming action that manifests itself electively on the bulbar centers and especially on the respiratory centers, coughing and vomiting.

For these activities, the drug preparations are used in therapy, alone or in combination, in cough and whooping cough sedative, antiasthmatic and antiemetic potions, which also gives a pleasant aroma.

Dandelion

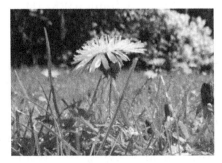

We should all be acquainted with what dandelions are, and Native Americans were quick to see how to utilize them medicinally.

For instance, did you realize that eating a dandelion salad (where you eat the leaves) can assist with mitigating a sensitive throat?

Did you likewise realize that dandelion is a diuretic and can, thusly, assist with passing pee? Simply drink some dandelion tea.

Echinacea

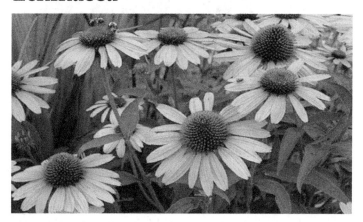

Plant Description

Lasting herbaceous plants 8-10 dm. high with round and hollow rhizome and somewhat ruddy stems. The leaves are basal and long petiolate, lanceolate with 3-5 veins with firm hairs. The assortment Angustifolia owes its name to the thin leaves, while the purpurea has leaves with more extensive pages. The inflorescences are framed at the middle by rounded blossoms and at the fringe by ligulati purple blossoms collapsed down in Angustifolia; more even in purpurea. The natural products are achenes.

Properties

Otherwise called purple echinacea, this is an exemplary Native American medication that is utilized to fortify the resistant framework, battle contaminations and fever. It is likewise utilized as a sterile and general treatment.

The extraordinary interest in the properties of echinacea gets from its capacity to enact the phagocytic activity of lymphocytes and reinforce the particular safe framework, of grown-ups and kids. The instrument of activity is communicated through an expansion in leukocytes, specifically, polymorphonuclear granulocytes (or neutrophils) and monocytes-macrophages of the reticuloendothelial framework, used to phagocyte (eat) destructive unfamiliar specialists (microorganisms, growths, and so forth. The plant likewise contains flavonoids, (for example, luteolin, kaempferol, quercetin, apigenin); caffeic corrosive subsidiaries (echinacoside, chlorogenic corrosive), cicoric corrosive, polyenes, alkylamides and fundamental oil. Specifically, echinacoside performs anti-toxin and bacteriostatic activity, ready to hinder the replication of microbes hard to control, while echinacea gives the plant calming corticosimilar properties.

At long last, the presence of cicoric corrosive and caffeic corrosive perform an antiviral activity, for example, to upset the infiltration of the infection in sound cells. A normal admission permits forestalling (particularly in periods when our body is dependent upon more prominent pressure) and treating the side effects of colds like fever, contaminations of the respiratory framework (cold, hack) and urinary framework (cystitis). For outer use, echinacea is additionally utilized for the readiness of treatments and salves for the skin, immunostimulant, defensive, mitigating, if there should arise an occurrence of scars, blister, ulcers, dermatitis overall. The recuperating property depends on the capacity of the plant to speed up tissue recovery and confine the disease.

Contraindications of Echinacea

Echinacea has not many incidental effects. Its immunostimulant activity makes it contraindicated in patients on immunosuppressive treatment (transfers, immune system illnesses).

Eucalyptus

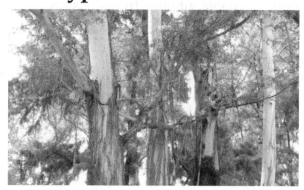

Plant Description

The fast-growing evergreen tree (reaches 20 m in 6-7 years), in Australia, land of origin, can exceed 90 m. The trunk has smooth, ash-gray bark, which detaches into thin, elongated plates. The wood is reddish. In eucalyptus globulus, the young leaves are opposite, blue in color, while the adult leaves are alternate, dark green, scythe-shaped and hard. The flowers are usually grouped in flower buds, more or less numerous. The fruit is a woody capsule, hard, wrinkled and covered with wax. The seeds are numerous and very small. The whole plant has an aromatic smell and bitter taste.

Properties

Eucalyptus leaves contain an essential oil, particularly rich in eucalyptol, terpenes (pinene, camphene, phellandrene); aldehydes; polyphenols (gallic acid, ferulic acid, gentisic acid); flavonoids (rutoside, hyperoside) and tannins. These active ingredients give the plant a balsamic, fluidifying and expectorant action of catarrhal secretions of the respiratory tract. Moreover, due to the presence of essential oil, eucalyptus has an antibacterial and antiseptic action very effective for urogenital tract diseases in case of cystitis, leucorrhoea and candidiasis, for which it is also recommended by virtue of its deodorant action. For cosmetic use, eucalyptus preparations exert a good antiseptic and healing action on purulent skin infections and soothing burns. Very suitable for cleansing skin and oily hair, to which it restores shine.

Contraindications

Eucalyptus essential oil, when used in large quantities, can lead to nausea, vomiting and diarrhea. It is therefore not recommended for use during pregnancy and while breastfeeding. It may also cause dermatitis and skin irritation in sensitive individuals.

Elderflower

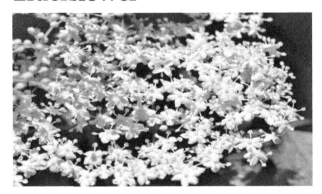

Elderflowers can be eaten in a variety of ways: jelly, syrup and tea are among the most popular.

The leaves, twigs, roots and stems cannot be safely consumed because they are toxic.

The elderflower extract is what is used for medicinal purposes. In particular, the extract can be used as a treatment for:

- Sweating
- Bleeding
- Bronchitis
- Constipation
- Colds
- Flu
- Common cold

Fennel

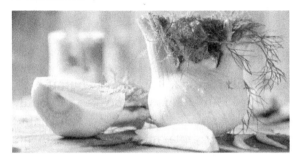

Fennel Description

Crisp and pleasantly fragrant, fennel is perhaps one of the most present vegetables on the tables of the Mediterranean area. The best climate for its cultivation is temperate but more prone to heat than cold. In Italy it is grown more or less everywhere, especially in the Centre and South, where it is widely used at the end of the meal, to aid digestion. There is also a variety of wild fennel.

Properties and Benefits

Fennel is best known for its digestive properties, but it is a friend of the entire gastrointestinal system. Fennel has the ability to prevent the formation of intestinal gas and contains anethole, a substance capable of acting on painful abdominal contractions. Fennel also has purifying properties, particularly for the liver and blood. It also has anti-inflammatory properties; it is composed mainly of water; among the minerals the most present is potassium; it contains vitamin A, vitamin C and some vitamins of the B group. It is fairly rich in flavonoids. It provides very few calories.

Curiosity about Fennel

Fennel is recommended in the diet for nursing women. It is said to facilitate milk production. In reality, however, fennel contributes above all to make its taste more pleasant.

Parthenium

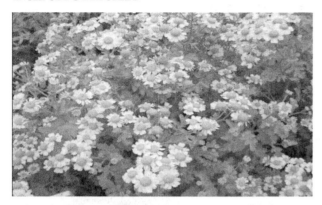

Plant Description

The Parthenium (Tanacetum parthenium), is a plant of the family of Composites. In Italy, depending on the place, it is known by the names of amarella, amareggiola, matricale, and maresina and marga grass. The plant has an erect and pubescent stem and can reach up to 70 centimeters in height. The leaves have a petiole and the flowers are very small and similar to tiny daisies. It is a perennial herb, little cultivated, but often present in the fields. It is about 80 centimeters high with a penetrating and unpleasant smell.

Properties

Parthenium is known for its anti-inflammatory properties. In particular, parthenium has a remarkable activity in migraine headaches, especially those defined vasomotor, in which there is an alternation of stimuli on the blood vessels that leads to vasoconstriction and subsequent vasodilation. This causes a deformation of the walls of the vessels themselves, which thus press on the nearby nerve endings, triggering pain, which can become increasingly excruciating due to the concomitant production of mediators that enhance the painful signal. The elements of the plant that contain the active ingredients are the aerial parts, especially the leaves, whose balsamic period, in which the concentration of active medicinal substances is maximum, is just before flowering. The main substances contained in Parthenium are flavonoids, sesquiterpenes, polyphenols, among which the most important for the medicinal activity of the plant is the parthenolide: these substances have the ability to reduce the contraction of smooth muscles and its excitability. This explains the use, since ancient times, of the Parthenium, which is a useful remedy for dysmenorrhea and migraine headaches. Some studies have also shown hypotensive properties, antispasmodic at the level of the digestive tract, also for the action on smooth muscles. It would also have, as a consequence, a mild tranquilizing effect that would facilitate sleep if the plant is taken in the evening. Its anti-inflammatory action also has a good soothing effect at the level of joint pain, including those resulting from rheumatoid arthritis.

Contraindications of Parthenium

Following the intake of Parthenium may appear allergic dermatitis and ulcerations of the mucous membranes (in contact with the fresh plant and in predisposed subjects), vomiting, diarrhea, headache, insomnia. Avoid in case of gastritis, ulcer, and hypersensitivity to one or more components. Not to be confused with Tanaceto (Tanacetum vulgare, sin. Chrysanthemum Vulgare), whose flowers were used in folk medicine as an anthelmintic remedy, now abandoned due to the presence of an essential oil rich in tuione, neurotoxic and abortive, it is contraindicated when taking serotonergic drugs (for example antidepressants). Do not administer to those who are allergic to composites. Prolonged use is not recommended, the prescription should be made by the doctor.

Feverwort

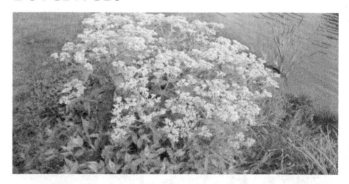

Description

Another fever remedy that is also used for general pain, itching and joint stiffness. It can be ingested like tea or chewed or crushed by a paste-like ointment or poultice. It is a plant of the Composite family that can reach up to one meter in height, with white flowers smelling vanilla. Native to the humid regions of North America, it has also been cultivated in Europe.

Plant Drugs, which is the part of the plant containing the highest concentration of active ingredients, used to prepare T.M., is the aerial part of the fresh flowering plant. It contains tannin, flavonoids (eupatorine), which have cytotoxic properties, triterpenes and phytosterols that cause bruising of the eye globes.

Indications

Indicated in flu-like febrile syndromes with the acme of fever at 7-9 a.m., sneezing, retrosternal night cough, eye globe pain and conjunctival hyperemia, facial bone pain, contusive myalgia, bone pain "as from broken bones" and need to change position in bed continuously.

Flaxseed

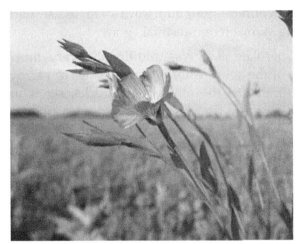

Flaxseed has also been used to treat kidneys.

Flaxseeds can also be consumed in any way you see fit, as long as they are not eaten raw or unripe. The best way to consume them is in powder form, or at least when dry.

Ginger

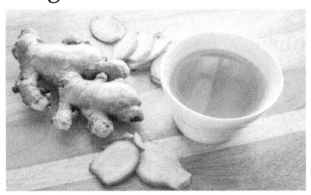

Description

Ginger (Zingiber officinale) is a perennial herbaceous plant of the family Zingiberaceae. Much used in cooking, it has some anti-inflammatory and digestive properties that make it useful for the stomach and heart. Ginger is very appreciated in cooking as a spice and by the food industry as a valuable flavoring (with ginger, for example, is produced the drink known as ginger ale), but it also has interesting medicinal properties. In commerce, it is found in the form of fresh or dried root, reduced to powder or extract or as candied ginger using only the natural sugar of its root. The dried ginger root powder is usually encapsulated and sold in handy tablets. There is not yet a consensus on dosage, but most doctors prescribe 500 mg to 1000 mg of ginger per day.

Properties of Ginger

Ginger is used as a natural anti-inflammatory and digestive aid and is among the most effective anti-inflammatory and antivertigo medicines. Ginger can be used to treat ailments such as motion sickness, seasickness, morning nausea, etc. Its antiemetic properties seem to reside locally on the walls of the stomach and intestine. In traditional Far Eastern medicine, ginger is used in the treatment of osteoarthritis, flu, as a heart stimulant, as a protective agent of the gastric mucosa. Thanks to its antibiotic properties, ginger is a valuable ally for the stomach, intestine, heart and circulatory system. Ginger essential oil is also rich in important properties. In fact, it is anti-inflammatory, invigorating, pain-relieving, digestive, antiviral and aphrodisiac; ginger is also useful against halitosis: in fact, it can be helpful to sip hot water boiled for 10 minutes with fresh ginger, a remedy that promotes digestion and counteracts the accumulation of toxins and bacterial fermentation.

Sumac

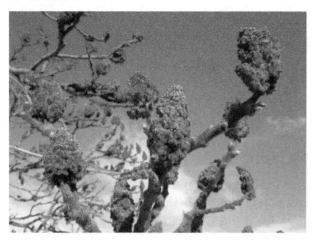

Sumac is excellent for treating colds, fevers and sore throats. To get these benefits, you need to prepare Sumac tea. Simply pick several bunches of berries and crush them lightly, soak them in a jug of cold water overnight, strain the mixture to remove the berries, and enjoy!

It's that simple. The pain won't go away completely, but you will feel almost instant relief and that's better than nothing.

Yarrow

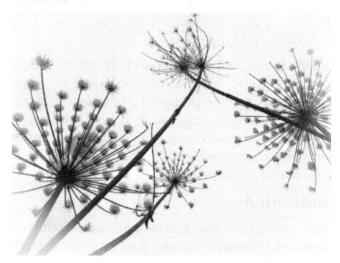

Yarrow is broad all through the world and was first used to incredible impact by the antiquated Greeks, who utilized it to stop inordinate draining by applying the leaves straightforwardly. They likewise took the juice from the yarrow and blended it in with water. This combination was then devoured straightforwardly to assist with treating stomach or intestinal agony.

The Cherokee clan was additionally very much aware of the solid restorative properties of yarrow and, similar to the antiquated Greeks, set it up principally as a tea. Essentially add a teaspoon of dried yarrow to some water, bubble for 10 minutes, strain the leaves and drink.

What's more, the Cherokee clan applied yarrow straightforwardly to the skin to assist with treating dry skin, skin inflammation and fresh injuries.

Part IV

~

Herbalism Encyclopedia & Apothecary II

Herbs of Wealth and Power

There are several herbs that are exceptionally valuable for wealth and power. They can be found around the world and are said to have been used by ancient Egyptians, Chinese herbalists, and Native American Indians. Here are some interesting facts about these herbs:

❖ The Romans considered fennel essential in their diet and even held public games of Fennel, a sporting event with twelve different events such as jumping with a rod or bending down over a sack of fennel.

❖ Chervil is often used in pickles because it is tasty-tasting without being too potent and can be added to salads also.

❖ Ginseng root tea has been consumed for thousands of years, from China to Central America.

❖ Licorice is the root of a plant and can be found in tea, candy, gum, and even cough drops.

❖ Anise is best known for its licorice flavor but it also was used to preserve foods like fish, vegetables, and cheese.

❖ Mint is one of the most popular herbs today. It can be found in candies, gum, toothpaste, and many dishes like lamb chops.

❖ Cinnamon has been imported from India for over a thousand years as a spice. This spice was so valuable that war was waged over it.

❖ Clove is one of the most highly prized spices. It was regarded as a holy spice by the ancient Egyptians and Greeks. Is hot, warming, and intoxicating. It helps with repelling negativity.

❖ Coriander was a valuable commodity among the Romans and was thought to be capable of curing snake bites, earache, and melancholy.

❖ Lavender is sweet and cleansing. It helps with nervousness, anxiety, restlessness.

❖ Cedarwood is sharp and inspiring. It helps with grounding and protection.

❖ Mint is cooling and refreshing. It helps with emotions of anger, frustration, nervousness, and sadness.

❖ Patchouli is spicy and grounding. It helps with protection from evil spirits and attracts good fortune in business ventures.

❖ Bay leaves are cleansing and refreshing to the mind. They attract strength from friends or family that want to help you achieve your dreams or goals.

❖ Sage is warming and vibrant. It helps with nerve pain, headaches, and muscle aches.

❖ Rosemary is stimulating and strengthening the mind. It helps with blood circulation, memory, and focus.

❖ Thyme is cleansing and sweet. It helps with fear of success or failure, fear of change, anxiety as well as insomnia.

❖ Lotus has a spiritual energy that helps one rest in peace within herself or himself; a symbol of purity, self-love, and self-acceptance which is essential for prosperity in all aspects of life. It also brings cosmic balance to the energies within the home or business environment before prosperity can be achieved within it. The lotus pond is a symbol of prosperity; the lotus blossom is a symbol of luxury and wealth; the lotus flower represents self-love and allows one to be at peace with himself or herself.

❖ Lucky Bamboo is used in mourning ceremonies and rituals. This herb will help bring good fortune and luck in all areas of life, such as gambling, money, success, health, relationships, thoughts, etc.

❖ Marigold is symbolic of abundance in all areas of life; it relates to financial prosperity. Used in ceremonies for banishing evil spirits from the home or business environment.

❖ Mullein has been used to alleviate pain and fever associated with sickness or injuries. It has also been used as a medicinal herb to aid in the healing of those with liver disorders. Mullein is used in ceremonies for prosperity. It will help bring good fortune and luck in all areas of life, such as gambling, money, success, health, relationships, thoughts, etc.

❖ Turmeric is used to cleanse the home or business environment from evil spirits or negative energies. It has been known to bring wealth and good fortune into homes that it is placed in.

❖ Yarrow flowers are used for attracting wealth and bringing good fortune into one's business ventures.

Herbs for Healing

There are thousands of healing herbs that can be used in different types of health problems. There are different kinds of herbs depending on the symptoms and condition you suffering from. Some herbs for healing include chamomile, dandelion root and ginseng.

These all have many medicinal properties that help with rejuvenating physical and spiritual health. Probably the most famous herb is Turmeric because it is a very effective treatment against Alzheimer's disease, inflammation, arthritis, cancer, diabetes-related diseases, and dental health issues. It also helps in reducing inflammation of skin after burns or injuries.

Bleeding wounds, cuts, and scrapes can be treated effectively with plantain seeds. Plantain seeds contain a number of vitamins and minerals that help boost the immune system. Another amazing herb that is used for healing is aloe vera. This herb has been used in Chinese medicines for thousands of years. It helps in treating burns, internal bleeding, toothache and sores on the lips, skin irritation, and inflammations.

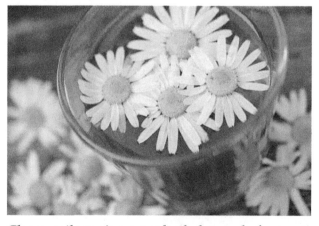

Chamomile tea is a great herbal remedy for treating bloating caused by gas and other stomach problems such as heartburns etc. There are many more herbs for healing. Some ancient herbs such as Ginseng and Ginkgo Biloba help to reduce cognitive problems, improve memory, concentration and increases mindfulness.

Garlic is also a very powerful medicinal herb that is used to treat cold-related illnesses, heart diseases, infections, etc. Ginger has been used in traditional Chinese medicine for years to treat muscle pain and other body pains that come with aging.

Valerian helps to calm down the nerves. This amazing herb has been proven to be effective in treating insomnia by inducing lucid dreams.

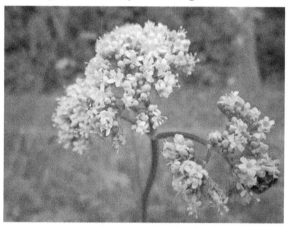

Cumin seeds are good for relieving diarrhea, stomach upset, and indigestion. On the other hand, dill seeds are good for relieving flatulence and intestinal upset.

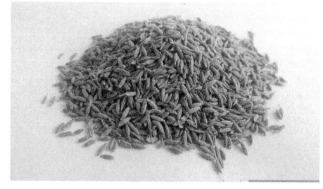

Cinnamon has been used as a spice for centuries so that it can help in easing irritability, depression, anxiety, and relieving coughs. Ginger is effective in treating nausea which is mostly caused by the use of some medications.

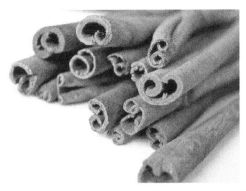

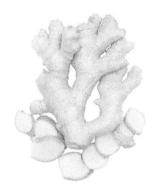

Eucalyptus Oil: This one's easy. Eucalyptus oil contains numerous properties which are known to help with ailments from respiratory to skin conditions. The oil has been used in healing for centuries and is still a frequently prescribed remedy within many countries including the UK, Canada, Australia, South America, and New Zealand. A few drops of this potent oil can help unblock congestion in your airways and boost your immune system.

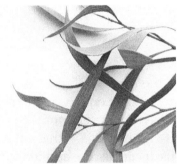

Ginger Root: The ginger plant is a perennial climbing herb that produces rhizomes and roots. It grows on other plants and can grow up to as high as 1.5 meters with lush green leaves that are spotted with reddish or yellowish-brown spots. The root has been used medicinally for centuries and contains numerous spicy oils and volatile oils which have profound healing properties, the most notable of which is gingerol which is widely known to help reduce inflammation in the body. Ginger's medicinal properties range from an internal analgesic to reduce pain in general, an anti-inflammatory, a nerve stimulant, to the treatment of nausea and morning sickness.

Hibiscus Tea: The hibiscus flower has been used for numerous health treatments. The flowers are rich in vitamin C, and the leaves contain other essential nutrients. The flower is most commonly used to make a tea with a vaguely fruity flavor, but can also be used to create jams or jellies. This unique fruit contains several phytochemicals that are known to stimulate circulation and reduce high blood pressure. In addition, the hibiscus is known to contain antioxidants that are capable of fighting free radicals, helping protect your body from many ailments including cancer.

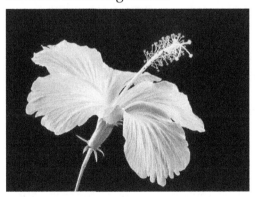

Lemon Balm: This plant contains numerous essential oils that have been used in medicinal treatments for centuries, most commonly for headaches. However, the herb has been recognized to possess anti-inflammatory, antispasmodic, antibacterial, antiviral, and sedative properties. It also contains compounds that have been shown to help the brain repair itself; specifically, the compound rosmarinic acid may be useful in helping repair damage caused by degenerative diseases such as Alzheimer's or dementia.

All these herbs are effective in healing illnesses when harvested from their natural source and prepared in the right way.

Herbs for Protection, Good Luck and Fertility

Herbs are an overlooked tool in our everyday lives. They can be used for protection, good luck, and fertility. This list of herbs is not exhaustive but should get you started.

Catnip: Use the catnip leaves for purification and protection from negative energies (similar to sage). The flowers are associated with love, luck and fertility (this can also be done with lavender). Cats will probably be attracted to the smell of catnip so this herb might not work if you have a problem with mice or other pests that come when they smell food (or something else in your house).

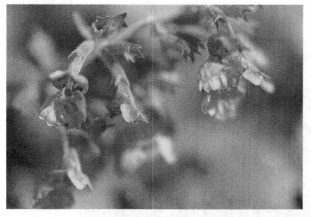

Lavender: The flowers are used for relaxation, protection from negative energy (like a sage), and fertility. There is even folklore that someone wearing lavender received their lover's love note in the mailbox that day. Applying lavender to the heart assists with purification as well as protection against negative spirits and bad luck (located around or in your home).

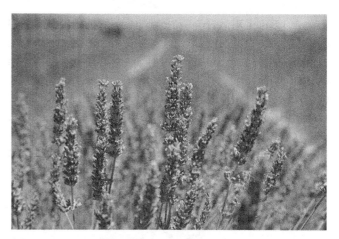

Mugwort: A powerful purifier of negative energy (like sage). Use the leaves to burn "as incense" for protection from negative energy and banishing bad luck. Burn the leaves in a ceremony or sacral bath when there is "something" that needs to be released. Mugwort can also be applied topically for healing and cleansing the aura (think of a Sage/Palm/Frankincense blend). Don't know what to use mugwort with yet? Try placing a few drops of oil in your pocket or purse. Both elements release negative energy. The oil will release negative energy if you happen to walk into an area where there are mice. Mugwort should help to purify the area around you. If you come across a mouse or rat, place a few leaves in your pocket and see if they drive the critters away.

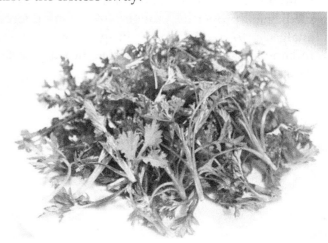

Mugwort/Mint: This combination is common in healing ceremonies as it aids the mind with its mental cleansing abilities. The infusion of these herbs can be used to purify negative energy and banish bad luck.

Sage: Both leaves and flowers are used to carry negativity away, protect from negative spirits, and cleanse your aura (see lavender for further details). Sage is also said to aid with fertility issues by balancing female hormones.

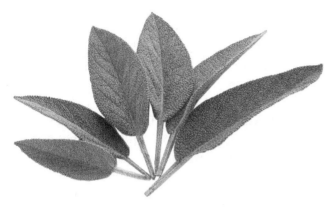

White Windsor: The leaves are used for purification and protection from negativity (like a sage). Burn the leaves in a ceremony or sacral bath when there is "something" that needs to be released. White Windsor can also be applied topically for healing and cleansing the aura (think of a Sage/Palm/Frankincense blend).

Yarrow: Yarrow is used as a purifying agent, an aid in meditation, and a heart tonic. It can be used to "cleanse" negative energies (like a sage). The flowers of this plant are used for love luck and fertility (this can also be done with lavender).

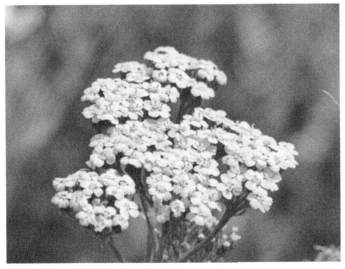

Valerian: The root is used for purification (like a sage). Valerian can also be used to enhance the

contraction of the uterus (either during pregnancy or as a preventive measure). Use the root as an infusion in a sacral bath. A common way of using valerian is by placing 1 ounce of dried roots in 1 cup of boiling water and steep for 10 minutes; strain out the roots and drink this infusion.

Yarrow/Valerian: Place 1 ounce of dried yarrow roots in 1 cup boiling water and steep for 10 minutes; strain out the roots and drink this infusion. The addition of valerian greatly increases its effectiveness as it helps to balance female hormones.

Yarrow/Valerian/Squawvine: Place 1 ounce of dried yarrow roots, 1 ounce of dried valerian roots, and 1 ounce of dried squawvine in 1 cup boiling water and steep for 10 minutes; strain out the roots and drink this infusion. The addition of squawvine greatly increases effectiveness as it helps to balance female hormones while also aiding infertility.

Goldenseal: Find a tincture or glycerin extract (it's a lot more concentrated) and use this herb to help with "hot flashes" associated with menopause. It is also used for purification (like sage).

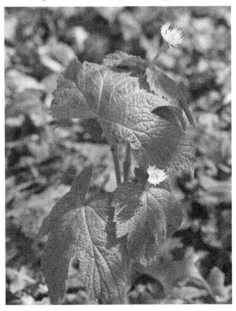

Kava Kava: The root is used in ceremonies. It aids in purification by effectively "clearing" a space of negative influences. It is also used as a pleasant alternative to alcohol with a numbing effect on the tongue and cheeks similar to peppermint candy.

Elder: The flowers are used for purification (like sage). Elder is also used as an anti-inflammatory for arthritis and other joint problems. Try placing some leaves in an organic hemp bag or use them as an infusion (see valerian).

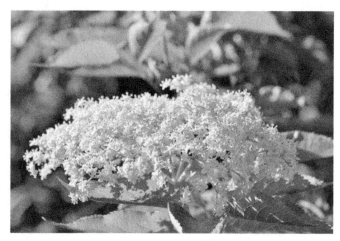

Rue: Place 1 ounce of rue in 1 cup boiling water; steep for 10 minutes; strain out the roots and drink this infusion. Ripe rue berries are poisonous and should not be used. Rue is used to purifying negative energy and to protect you (or space) from bad luck. It is also used for fertility concerns.

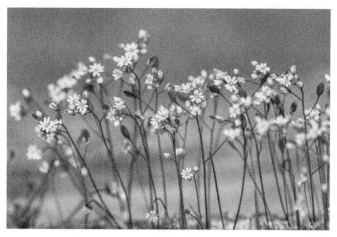

Sage/Mugwort/Lavender: These herbs are best when combined in a sacral bath (1 cup dried herbs in 2 cups boiling water). Don't know what to use mugwort with yet? Try placing a few drops of oil in your pocket or purse. Both elements release negative energy. The oil will release negative energy if you happen to walk into an area where there are mice. Mugwort should help to purify the area around you. If you come across a mouse or rat, place a few leaves in your pocket and see if they drive the critters away.

Sage/White Windsor: These herbs are best when combined in a sacral bath (1 cup dried herbs in 2 cups boiling water). White Windsor is the best choice for completing this combination.

Herbs for Love and Beauty

In ancient times, all kinds of herbs were used to increase the attraction between two people and make them fall in love. Some examples of these plants are basil, rosemary, lemongrass, lavender, and garlic. These plants were exchanged as gifts because they had significant effects on feelings. To enhance attractiveness in general these plants usually have a red or purple flower which is why the term "herb of love" was coined.

In ancient Greece, herbs were consumed to improve one's appearance. Dioscorides prescribes violets and roses to be added to wine and drank in small amounts. Pliny the Elder also describes some concoctions containing violets.

Lavender was used by the Ancient Greeks in their ointments because of its calming effect on the body; it was also used as a perfume in the Middle Ages. In those times it was thought that lavender helped you sleep better when placed under your pillow which led to giving lavender for love.

In the Middle Ages, rosemary was more commonly used to enhance love and attraction between partners. As with lavender, it was thought that the vapor from the plant could help you sleep better in bed which led to giving rosemary for love. The reason people used rosemary was because of its taste. The taste reminded people of honey which meant sweet things were associated with it. Because of this association rosemary was sometimes used as a spice in dishes instead of cinnamon which had a more bitter taste.

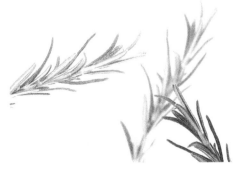

Lemongrass had an obvious odor that one could identify as lemon, hence was often added to

perfume mix on its own or mixed with other floral scents such as roses and violets, etc.

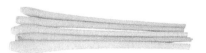

Garlic has an odor that is similar to that of other members of the onion family like leeks and onions. According to ancient Rome, it could increase love by attracting the opposite sex.

Basil and marjoram are used to calm nerves and induce sleepiness which is why basil was often consumed in bedtime drinks to help you fall asleep and have a good night's sleep. In addition, basil is used in many types of food as a garnish; for this reason, it was considered a common herb.

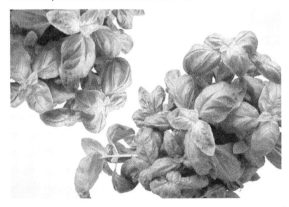

In ancient Rome, rosemary was recognized for its stimulating aroma which reminded people of their loved ones who were far away or dead, hence giving rosemary as an offering for love back home was common practice. Rosemary was also used as a seasoning instead of cinnamon which had a more bitter taste.

In English folklore, rosemary was considered to be a magic herb and protected humans against witches and spells. It was also associated with the Virgin

Mary so it could protect against evil spirits and bad dreams. Around mid-January people would burn rosemary leaves to ward off evil spirits. People also believed that if you put it in your socks you would see fairies at night when you are asleep or if you hang some above your door you will see an angel during the night or if hung above a baby's bed then the child will become smarter (this one is ironic because rosemary contains camphor which is toxic).

In olden Europe, the red lily of the valley was one of the most common herbs used in love potions. It has a sweet scent that is similar to violets and is known as an aphrodisiac and is thought to enhance pleasure and relaxation. In addition, it was also used as a scent in love potions because it reminded people of roses which were associated with love.

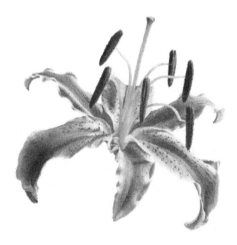

Myrtle has a sweet odor but it can be compared to a red apple smell. It was used externally because the skin absorbs it well and from ancient times up until modern days, people have applied myrtle oil on their skin and applied on their feet to help fight infections such as athlete's foot.

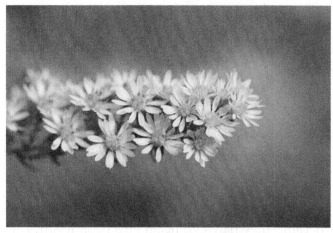

Violet is traditionally associated with love and was used in love potions because of its sweet scent. The flavor is very similar to that of strawberries and strawberries are known as a symbol of love in most cultures. It can also have a narcotic effect which provides people with feelings of relaxation and pleasure and this is why violet has been used as an antidepressant since the Middle Ages.

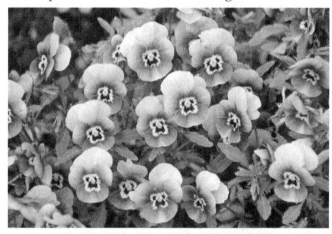

Tansy has a strong smell that could be compared to the smell of musk. This herb was often added to magical incense, love potions, or magic powders. The reason for adding tansy to such things was because it was said to scare away evil spirits from people and their homes better than other herbs such as basil or lemongrass, etc. It was also used for its healing properties because it has a strong antibiotic effect and is known to destroy bacteria and viruses.

Herbs for Special Purposes

Ginkgo Biloba

One benefit of Ginkgo Biloba is that it helps maintain healthy blood circulation in our veins and arteries, which would help with memory problems (reduced ability to think) as well as headaches. A possible disadvantage would be that it can cause nausea in some people if taken on an empty stomach; it might also interact with other medications.

Green tea is another popular herbal supplement, with numerous reports of it being effective for weight loss and the prevention of many cancers. In addition, green tea is a very rich source of antioxidants. A disadvantage would be that it can reduce the effectiveness of other medications; also, for some people, it can cause constipation. There are many green tea extracts available but these are standardized extracts; in general, the higher the concentration, the less you will need to take.

One commonly used herb is garlic (due to its very high antioxidant levels). One possible bad effect would be that it can interact with other medications.

It has been suggested that alcohol may be effective in reducing the symptoms of Parkinson's disease and is possibly beneficial in treating Alzheimer's disease. A downside to using alcohol medicinally is the potential adverse effects on those who drink too much, especially if they are taking medications that include alcohol as an ingredient.

Other commonly used herbs for their antioxidant or detoxifying effects include green tea, St. John's wort (Hypericum perforatum), black tea (Camellia sinensis), and red wine (Culicis arvensis).

The most commonly used herbs for the treatment of digestive disorders are peppermint (Mentha x Piperita), lemon balm (Melissa officinalis), artichoke leaf (Cynara scolymus) and black cumin seed (Nigella sativa). However, some of the herbs may cause allergic reactions in some people. Another commonly used herb is ginger root (Zingiber officinale). It has been shown in pharmaceutical trials to reduce nausea caused by chemotherapy. Ginger root may interact with other medications; however, the dose used was very high, and this potential interaction was not tested by pharmaceutical manufacturers.

Boswellia serrata is a common ingredient in herbal anti-inflammatory preparations for the treatment of arthritis. It has also been shown to reduce symptoms of numerous allergies, including asthma. However, the herb was effective only when taken with certain medications; other anti-inflammatory herbs that do not include Boswellia Serrata were not effective.

Another commonly used herb is Devil's claw (Harpagophytum procumbens). In one study, 82% of patients showed significant improvement in their symptoms while taking this herb for 2-3 months. The herb also reduced pain and stiffness in those with osteoarthritis; however, it did not work for all patients.

An increase in the use of herbal remedies is partly due to their availability. The most common ways to use herbs are through teas, which can be readily prepared at home.

Feverfew (Tylecodon grandiflorus) is a common herb that is used for the treatment of migraine headaches. The herb contains parthenolide, which inhibits the release of serotonin. A disadvantage of this herb is that it has been reported to cause liver damage in some patients; however, a common form of feverfew does not contain parthenolide. Another commonly used herb for migraines is butterbur (Petasites hybridus).

Part V

~

Native American Herbalism and Alchemy

Introduction

Native American herbology has been around for over 100 years, and it is considered the oldest form of medicine still practiced today. The main goal of this way of life and medicine is to bring the human body back into harmony and balance with nature. It does so through a variety of techniques and methods, including herbalism, tonics, dieting, and even spiritual practices. Some people say that Native American herbology dates back to some of the first healing ceremonies recorded in history, but it didn't become mainstream until around 15 years ago, when modern medicine was beginning to have a negative impact on the overall health of our planet.

Native American herbology tends to use herbal medicines and practices instead of synthetic chemicals like traditional medicine does. Natural and organic herbs are used in these formulas to give back the body what it lacks in any given situation.

Folk medicine is considered a type of medicine that uses plants for healing instead of modern drugs and treatments. Here the word "folk" means "people," so folk medicine is basically the same as Native American herbalism even though it might not be as mainstream as most people think.

"When the earth has no power, nothing is alive. Man is a dead thing. It is when the earth is full of life that man will be complete." Chief Seattle (1854).

"The white man who touches the green leaves of Indian country has been poisoned by contact with something sacred. The Indian knows this very well and does not like to see it." Vine Deloria Jr. (1969).

When you've done your research into Native American herbology, you'll understand why it is such a beneficial way of dealing with many health problems, including hair loss, body aches, arthritis, and more. It has been practiced for centuries by many different tribes across the US. These herbs are used as remedies for a variety of reasons, including helping to lose weight, increasing sexual function, reducing stress, and more.

Folk medicine or herbal remedies have been used in this country since around the 17th century. The Native Americans were the first people on this earth that had extensive knowledge of how to heal themselves with plants from their surroundings. The first thing you would do is cut a branch off from a plant and chew on it to see if it had any healing powers. You could then drink the water the branch came from, and you would have a sense of relief and well-being after that.

Another thing that people should consider when they are looking at Native American herbology recipes is to know what they are dealing with. The ingredients used in these formulas are very safe for most people, with no side effects. You can also safely take them by themselves by doing a blend of them in a healthy meal, like soup or something similar.

Native American Diagnosing Ailments

Native Americans were the first to develop and introduce the idea of diagnosing and treating ailments, as well as understanding natural healing processes. Native Americans have used various methods throughout history for healing the mind, body, and spirit.

1. Traditional Healing – wordless chants that include visualization of a vision or a plant
2. Spiritual Healing – performing rituals such as sweat lodges or fire cleansings to migrate spiritual energy in order to bring balance in all aspects of life
3. Mind/Body Medicine – using holistic practices with herbal remedies or practices which help clear up physical ailments through mental guidance without prescription drugs
4. Praying Medicine – using certain substances to heal a person of disease or illness through prayer

It is believed that Native Americans were able to understand the medicinal qualities of a plant prior to testing it on themselves. They first made sure the plant was not poisonous as they gathered herbs, roots, and water from natural sources. "They talked in their own language about which plants would work for them." Native American traditional healers used prayer and chants wordlessly. Envisioning their ailments away was another way prayer became a major component of healing. By chanting wordless, Native Americans believed that they could visualize the problem leaving with the chant as well as clear their mind for it to happen.

In addition to chanting, Native Americans also performed sweat lodges and fire cleansings. These rituals were used to clear sickness, disease, and other health problems in order for the body to heal itself. Fire cleansings were very common among the native peoples of America. They purified a room by starting a fire then burning sage and cedar over the ashes of the fire.

There are different types of prayer such as Smudging (clearing a space), Sweat Lodges (a ceremony in which one or more people bring their health concerns in front of a fire), and Fire Cures (to cleanse one's spirit).

Smudging was the most popular form of prayer, which involved burning a mixture of herbs over a fire. The Smudging ceremony is done to bring good luck and protection. The Fire Cures was a cleansing they did by burning sage and cedar in the sacred room, bringing healing. Another way they cleared the room and purified the spirit was by using sweat lodges which involved having two fires: One inside and one outside near the door to invite good energy.

Overall, Native Americans were highly attuned to their surroundings as well as their surroundings' natural resources in order to better understand how they worked. They would use what they needed as well as what they had. By making their own medicines and using natural plants, Native Americans were able to gain a better understanding of these herbs and how they worked together.

Medicine beads—a prayer offering to the Great Spirit made into a necklace or bracelet to be worn.

Smoking medicine (medicine put in tobacco)—a prayer offering to the Great Spirit made into small sticks or packs of leaves which are then smoked.

Sacred pipes—sacred pipes are normally used by Native Americans by placing tobacco through the "smokebox" (a hollowed-out earth dish with smoke holes. In the early 19th century, this type of pipe was sometimes called a "peace-pipe.") It is then smoked in a circular motion, with each participant smoking it in turn.

Herbs for Arthritis

If you're one of the millions of people who suffer from arthritis, you know that the pain can make even simple tasks difficult. And while there are plenty of pharmaceutical options to help reduce inflammation and ease joint symptoms, sometimes it's just as effective (and far less expensive!) to turn to another type of herbal remedy.

In fact, many of the herbs traditionally used for joint pain are now recognized by the NIH as effective options to manage arthritis symptoms. You can find many of these herbs in herbal supplements or teas that you can order online, and make a tea or tincture at home.

Among the most effective herbal remedies for arthritis are astragalus, Boswellia, and devil's claw.

Astragalus is one of the most well-known herbs for arthritis—in fact; it's been used in China for thousands of years to treat all sorts of ailments, including inflammation. It is especially effective when used with other herbs like devil's claw since they work together to reduce pain and inflammation.

Dosage: You can find astragalus in dried root form at most Chinese pharmacies, or you can make your own tincture.

Boswellia is another herb that has been used for thousands of years to reduce inflammatory pain. It's available in most health food stores, but it can be difficult to find the extract (Boswellia serrata) over the counter. The recommended dosages are typically quite high.

Dosage: Boswellia extract is typically sold in capsules; these capsules may be very expensive, depending on where you buy them—here are some recommendations. For a lower-cost alternative, you can make your own tincture by making a 10:1 extract with alcohol, glycerin, and water.

Devil's claw is an herb that was once used as a pain reliever by indigenous people of Africa and Asia. When you purchase it in tincture form, it usually comes in 5 or 10% concentration, while most of the higher concentration prescription-strength products come in 30 to 60%. One reason this may be so is that the percentages are not exact; the 30% of products are actually much stronger than they appear on the label. This herb is a good choice for rheumatoid arthritis symptoms.

Dosage: The recommended dose of dried devil's claw root is 900 to 1,800 mg per day. An extract made from the plant has been proven effective in reducing the pain and inflammation that comes with arthritis. However, it seems very difficult to find any devil's claw extract produced in the US for a reasonable price; this extract is typically imported from Europe and costs upwards of $90 for 60 capsules (about two months' worth).

Luckily, you can make your own high-quality devil's claw tincture using these instructions.

I recommend taking one or two dropperfuls of the tincture three times a day. This is equivalent to about 1,800 mg. of the herb.

Another remedy with proven effectiveness is Boswellia extract, which has been shown to be an effective pain reliever for arthritis patients in clinical studies. It can be used by itself or used in combination with astragalus as described above. This herb comes in capsules, but it can also be made into a tincture at home. Here are some instructions on how to do this. You'll want to make enough tincture to last you several weeks for joint pain relief and keep it on hand if you have any flare-ups during that time.

Another remedy that can help reduce arthritis pain is capsaicin cream. Even though it may seem counterintuitive to apply a painful substance like pepper to an arthritic joint, the capsicum in the cream actually decreases pain and inflammation.

Dosage: Capsaicin cream comes in different percentages—the higher the percentage, the more painful it is going to be. Apply one of these creams twice a day for best results. The higher doses may also cause flushing and tingling of your skin, which only last for a few minutes and aren't harmful. Because it can be quite painful, I usually recommend trying it at a lower dose if you have any issues with flushing or itching.

Rosemary is another herbal remedy that has been proven to be effective for arthritis symptoms. You can buy dried rosemary in the spice section of your local grocery store, or you can make tea using this recipe. You'll want to take one teaspoon of the herb per cup of water for two cups of tea. If you choose rosemary as an option for arthritis, add a little lemon juice to counteract the bitterness.

In addition to these herbs individually, many other herbs have been proven effective as herbal remedies for arthritis—some are mentioned above and others are mentioned here. Keep in mind that most of the research on medicinal herbs has been conducted on extracts, not the whole herb. So, an herb may be effective when taken as an extract or tincture, but may not work as well when taken in a tea or food.

Facts about Native Medicine

If you are thinking about using native American medicine, it can be extremely helpful to think about the motivations behind your decision. Native American medicine is an incredibly personal choice and involves experimentation with different lifestyles, medicines, and spiritual rituals. For some people, that means a deep desire for change, in order to live a healthier or happier life.

For others who have used this form of treatment before and seen positive results, it may mean that they want to return to the person they were pre-recovery; someone who was not constantly struggling with addiction but happy and healthy because they took control of their own well-being. A logical step would be to consider looking for help from a native medicine specialist, but how do you know if western medicine is the right method for you?

The biggest benefit of a journey into Native American medicine is that it brings us closer to the nature around us. It gives us insights into the importance of our surrounding environment and it helps us to understand that we are not separate from the Nature, but an intrinsic part of it. The last thing that many people want to do when they are in recovery is a return to their addictions, even though they will always be with them in some form.

The fact is, some people who are in recovery are unable to find a happy, healthy lifestyle and return to their high school mentality and set of addictions. For others, being in recovery offers a holistic approach to life and the ability to be at peace with themselves.

This is why Native American Medicine is such an effective method of treatment in the United States today. It offers those who have been struggling with addiction or those who have been through the natural stages of life a positive way forward that does not involve alcohol or drugs as part of their lifestyle. It also shows them that they are not alone and that there are many ways of helping them to heal.

For those who are using drugs or alcohol to cover up their physical, mental, emotional, or spiritual pain, this healing can be very attractive and highly effective.

In order to start your journey with Native American medicine, it can be helpful to think about what you want out of the experience and how to ensure that your goals are met. It is often said that learning about our past is a way of avoiding going down the same path twice and it can help us to understand why we have made certain choices in life. This experience can help you to rediscover yourself after years of being lost and it will show you another way of life that you may not have known existed before.

In order to take the most benefit from Native American medicine, it is important to remember that it comes from the ancient wisdom of people who lived on the land that is now America, thousands of years ago. The belief was that people were woven into Nature and that the intrinsic relationship between humans and the land could only be healed by looking at what caused harm within both your body and soul.

The main way of healing was through ceremony, a process that involved different aspects such as fasting, chanting, medicinal herbs, and a positive attitude. The most important aspect of the ceremony was that it involved a whole community, in order to be as effective as possible. This could mean family, friends, other addicts who wanted to heal their bodies or minds, or even the natural surroundings themselves.

Today's medicine is a stripped-down version of what was used by Native Americans thousands of years ago and it can be used in the twenty-first century because it centers on the importance of balance in life. It involves identifying what is causing you pain both on an emotional and physical level and coming up with a plan that works for you to be able to identify when those issues arise in your life again.

In a world that is so fast-paced, it can be hard to find time to pause and reflect on your life. It can also be difficult for people in recovery to find a way forward when they are not sure what they want from their lives. Native American medicine offers the perfect option for both of these types of people because it can help you to rediscover yourself, learn about the positive aspects of nature and the importance of balance in your body and soul, and it can give you the stability that you need in order to get back on your feet after years of struggling with addiction.

Part VI

~

Essential Oils

Extractions and Essential Oils

Extracting is a wonderful thing. It's what allows us to very easily make things like tinctures, salves, and oils from herbs. It's through the process of extracting that we get the healing phytochemicals our bodies crave and that make herbs useful medicine.

This list is by no means a comprehensive picture of all the things you can do with plants, so please take it as an introduction to making medicinal preparations rather than a complete guide.

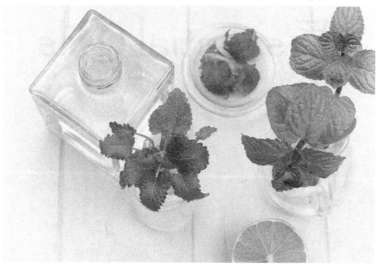

But what exactly is an extraction? An extraction is a technique where you put whole herbs into a liquid, and the plant's essential oils and phytochemicals are extracted. Extractions also involve drying out the herbs, so they retain their properties, but they are also safe to use, and you can add other ingredients to create new formulas.

Terms

There are a few terms that are useful to know about, especially if you want to use herbs as a healing agent.

Tonics

Tonics are usually taken in small doses and have effects on the body, but not necessarily a direct effect on disease. These can be used for overall conditioning or promotion of health.

Tonics do not have to be taken internally; they can be applied externally as well, for example, as an ointment for skin conditions or to promote general healing. Tonics can also be taken in the form of tea.

Tonic herbs are generally low in potency, and examples of them include marshmallow root, motherwort, and goldenseal root.

Herbal Teas

Herbal tea is made by steeping dried herbs in hot water. Herbal teas can be made from fresh herbs too, but dried is most common for use as a medicinal preparation. Herbal teas are often mixed with other herbs such as peppermint, chamomile, and lemon balm.

Herbal teas can be used topically in the form of a poultice or bath to soothe aches and pains, as well as to promote health. They can be taken as a tisane or infused in a cup of hot water. Some herbal teas, such as chamomile, can be useful for children with upset stomachs or upset, emotional states.

Decoction

Decoctions are made by simmering or boiling whole herbs in water. This is a great way of using herbs with high potency.

Infusions

Infusions are made by steeping the herbal material in hot water. They are usually done in whole food, such as fruit, and even chocolate or honey. Herbal infusions can be taken as teas or tinctures.

Tinctures

Tinctures are made by steeping dried herbs in alcohol for up to 90 days or until dry. Tinctures are usually used to preserve the phytochemicals in the herbs, although there are also tinctures that have been simply infused with alcohol that can be used. A tincture contains a much lower potency of herbal material than a tea or infusion.

Aromatherapy and Flower Essences

Flower essences are among the most popular home remedies for anxiety.

These remedies were founded by Edward Bach, a homeopath in England during the early 1900s, who was fascinated with the idea that flowers had healing properties. He did not believe in chemical medicine and even said, "In letting nature take its course, we are letting God take his." His aim was to find a way to heal people without using the medicine, which he believed led to a dependency on more and more drugs.

What he found is that when he placed a flower in a bowl of water and allowed it to sit overnight, the flower's energy would infuse the water. When taken internally, this water could treat what he called a "specific condition," such as fear or guilt.

A few drops of these flower essences are usually taken under the tongue four times daily (or as directed by an herbalist) and are supposed to change our vibration from fear to love through their unique vibrational frequencies.

Some people who experience synesthesia, in addition to experiencing the sense of a different color when they hear sounds, also see colored shapes and forms or get numbers as sounds. Others might have what is referred to as "visual sound," where they see words or words blended together while reading them.

Synesthetes often develop synesthesia later in life and are highly intelligent and creative individuals who can even use their unique abilities to help themselves solve puzzles. Synesthetes also tend to have an excellent imagination and an affinity for art.

Aromatherapy is the use of certain plant essences as medicine through their scent. These are also known as essential oils and are extracted using either distillation or expression. The word "aromatherapy" is a combination of the Greek word for aroma, "aroma" and the French word for therapy, "therapie."

Distillation involves steeping a plant in water and collecting its components that evaporate, which can then be used to make the essential oils. The process of distillation is extremely time-consuming and expensive, but is the most effective way of extracting essential oils.

Expression (also called "cold pressing") uses steam to extract the resin from the plant, which is then pressed and dried for storage. The concept behind the expression is very similar to that of distillation—where the plant's essence (essence meaning life force) is released into the steam so it can be collected and used if you suspect you might have some form of synesthesia or a sense of color, sound, etc.

Oils

Infused Oils

Infused oils are an excellent way to add flavor and depth to your cooking. The process is simple: You take high-quality oil like olive or canola, you put it in a jar, and then you fill the jar with ingredients like fresh rosemary and thyme leaves, which will give it flavor. Voilà! You've got infused oil that's ready for use.

How to Make Them

The process couldn't be easier or more foolproof! Just find your favorite herbs, chop them finely, pack them loosely into a clean glass jar (like these), and pour in the desired amount of oil (anywhere from ¼ cup to 2 cups) so there's plenty of space on top. This is normal.

You can make infused oils with any herb or combination of herbs, but a great place to start is rosemary and thyme. Here's an easy way to make your own rosemary-infused olive oil.

Select firm, hard-skinned ripe fruits of fresh rosemary plants from your garden. Do not use dried rosemary in infusing oils; it will not have the right amount of herbal taste or smell. (You can use dried herbs, whatever you prefer.) Place several sprigs of fresh rosemary into a jar (do not pack tightly; it needs room for the herbs to expand). Fill the jar with olive oil (between ¼ and 2 cups). Using any flavored olive oil will work; we like a fruity one for this particular recipe. You can use infused oil made from herbs such as rosemary or thyme straight from the garden, but in order to make sure there's enough flavor, you generally want to infuse oils for at least 7 days. After that, refrigerate the oil.

Essential Oils

Essential oils are natural, aromatic substances that come from plants. They're used widely in perfumery, aromatherapy, and alternative medicine as remedies for a wide range of ailments. A couple of people in the United States use them routinely to give themselves contact with the world around them, while others purchase them at local shops or online retailers.

What Are Essential Oils?

Essential oils are concentrated aromatic compounds that come from plants. Actually, they're often the most volatile chemical composition of a plant because their aroma is responsible for its reproduction and pollination. As such, plants make them in very small amounts and would only be able to provide for their needs by manufacturing more if they were cut or bruised. This also explains why some plants release much more essential oil when crushed or broken than others, although researchers have yet to determine why this is exactly the case.

Researchers are interested in essential oils for a variety of different uses. Some of the most common include aromatherapy, perfume, cologne production, food flavoring, and medicine. Essential oils are also used widely to create perfumes due to their pleasant aroma, but they're also an excellent way to make the air smell better when combined with other compounds. People can purchase essential oils from local merchants or online sellers, and they generally have a variety of scents from which to choose.

Why Do I Need Them?

Essential oils provide people with a variety of benefits that range from psychological to physical in nature. For instance, aromatherapy can be used to help relax your mind and body. Its effects are especially useful during times when you don't feel comfortable or at ease, but there is nothing wrong with feeling the need for some rest.

Similar to aromatherapy, essential oils can also improve your mood and make you feel more relaxed after a long, stressful day at work or study. This is especially ideal if you're not feeling motivated as soon as you step out into the world on a busy day, but its effects fade quickly, so it's best to take advantage of it while it's still present.

In addition to being used for aromatherapy, essential oils are also an excellent way to add flavor to your food. These compounds have unique tastes and scents that will complement your favorite food dishes in a number of different ways. You might also find that your food can taste better with the addition of these compounds, but this depends entirely on how you expect it to taste beforehand, so there's no point in not trying them out.

Essential oils, if consumed orally, can also be used as medicine to help reduce symptoms or cure an illness.

How to Use Essential Oils

By now, you're probably familiar with how essential oils are made and know that they derive from plants. The good news is that it's quite easy to use essential oils in your everyday life. They're also excellent as gifts because they provide a wide range of benefits and can be used for a variety of different purposes, such as perfume creation. To get started making essential oil products at home, it's possible to buy an inexpensive essential oil distillation kit that will allow you to create them at home without having to purchase commercial equipment.

Essential Oils and Their Properties

There are more than 7,000 different essential oils on the market that people can purchase from local merchants or online retailers. Each oil has a unique composition and purpose, which makes it possible for you to discover the best essential oils for your needs, but they all share a few common characteristics. They're generally potent, with most of them containing between 0.1–5% of their active components in their finished form, which makes them seem much stronger than they actually are. Additionally, there are many different ways to categorize essential oils based on their chemical makeup and test results.

For instance, some of them are classified as monoterpenes, while others are classified as sesquiterpenes, which are the most common types of essential oil, and they contain more than a hundred different compounds. These oils can have qualities that make them very strong or relatively weak based on their particular composition. Some examples of sesquiterpenes include rose, lavender, and sandalwood, but they all share similar properties that make them useful in perfumery products.

The chemical makeup is also important because some essential oils can be categorized as being either highly volatile or non-volatile, which affects their effectiveness during inhalation and oral consumption. This means that the vast majority of essential oils are very potent, and they're often classified by their volatile quality.

Oils with relatively low volatile qualities are believed to have properties that make them more effective as a gift for perfuming or as inhalation because of their ability to be absorbed into your body following inhalation. Many oils with low volatile qualities are believed to be safe when consumed orally because they're not considered highly toxic, but it's still important to check the product description before purchasing any essential oil in order to know exactly what you're getting. In fact, some oils can be very dangerous when swallowed, so it's always recommended that you only consume these oils by applying them topically or inhaling them through the nose.

Preparing Herbal Oils

Herbal oil is a tincture, liniment, or maceration of herbs that are made to be applied topically.

A liniment is a liquid preparation made by combining water and the essential oil of the herb in question. It can also contain alcohol to extract more of the constituents from the plant matter into the liquid. They're often used for arthritis pain relief, muscle spasms, sports injuries, or sore muscles. A tincture would then be a mixture of alcohol and water. An ointment is made by adding oil to the herbal mixture, which is then applied to the skin.

Herbal oil can be used as a beauty aid, body care product (such as a lotion) or hair care product (such as a conditioner).

Herbal oils can also be used in aromatherapy: Inhaling herbal oils through diffusion or massage. It's also used for applying them topically to soothe irritated skin or sore muscles. A good example of this would be using lavender for burns, chamomile for eczema, and peppermint for insect bites (since it's known to repel them).

Herbal oils can also be used in compressed by applying them to a cloth, then applying it to the affected area (such as a shoulder that's injured), or soaking a bandage in the herbal oil for treating wounds. They can also be used in bath additives or cataplasms (a type of plaster that's applied to the skin). Herbal oils are used for both external and internal ailments.

When using herbal oil on your skin, always apply the smallest amount possible. The herb content is very concentrated, and some may have side effects, such as irritation, which means you just need one drop to cover an entire affected area.

Another thing you'll want to do is make sure you have a way of extracting the essential oils before you start making the herbal oil.

Extracting the Essential Oils

You can use several methods for this. If you're using dried herbs, then just follow these instructions:

1. Place the herbs in a pot with a small amount of water. You want it to be enough to cover the dried herb by about an inch and a half. Bring this mixture to boil for 5–10 minutes (depending on how strong you want it). Then simmer the mixture for another 20–30 minutes (once again, depending on how strong you want it).
2. Remove from the liquid and let cool to room temperature. Strain it through a cheesecloth or a paper towel.

If you're making oils that will be applied topically or ingested, then you want to make sure the essential oils are extracted, so they remain in the oil instead of going into your body or being expelled through your lungs when inhaled. This is called essential oil extraction.

To do this, follow these directions:

1. Place one part herb, two parts grain alcohol (or 70 proof vodka). The herb can be dried or fresh, and the alcohol can be 70 proof or regular.
2. Let the mixture sit for at least 1 week at room temperature (a couple of days is even better).
3. Strain the mixture through a cheesecloth or a paper towel, and discard the herbs.
4. Use a reusable glass wide-mouth jar to store your oil. If you're storing it in a plastic container, it's best to use one that's not air-tight since the essential oils will absorb into the container over time.

The next time you need home remedies for a cold, flu, sore throat, joint pain or any other ailment, know that there are many ways to prepare herbal oils. You can create pills and lozenges from the herbs used in your remedies, make suppositories from the oils of fresh plants, use bath and bathing remedies as a quick aid for aches and pains, or boil herbs in oil so they can be infused into creams or lotions.

This guide provides instructions for each method. Learn how to make soap from an oil blend of rosemary, lavender, chamomile, and myrrh, or use a mix of olive oil and coconut oil as an all-purpose natural cleaner. Try a lavender wash to soothe the symptoms of a cold or treat a dry scalp with ginger and rosemary sanitizing hair tonic.

Herbal oils can be used all over the body — from head to toe. In fact, you have many options when it comes to using herbal oils for healing.

The benefits of herbal oil include its ability to be absorbed into the skin and muscles and its versatility in terms of where it can be applied. You can use oils as a moisturizer for dry or sensitive skin and for massage. Some herbal oil blends are intended to help with joint pain or stiffness in the neck, shoulders, or back.

Another benefit of herbal oils is their ease of application. You can simply rub them on the skin or mix them into bathwater. Many people find that these remedies help them relax as well as minimize aches and pains.

Making herbal oil blends is only one method of creating topical remedies. You can also make and use your own herbal oil or purchase ready-made options at a health food store or natural foods market. This guide includes suggestions of herbs that are good for treating a wide range of ailments, and it also gives information on the proper way to prepare them for use in healing remedies.

Herbal oils are essential tools for any herbalist. They provide you with a fast and effective means to use plants as natural medicines. Making herbal oils is also a great way to create the flavor that complements your herb blend recipes. Whether you are creating herbal oils for topical applications or using them in your cooking, they will help you take full advantage of the healing properties of plants.

Extractions

The use of essential oils dates back to over 3,000 years ago and is often attributed to Damaris. The extraction process for essential oils is a relatively simple process that does not require a lot of time or special equipment.

The first step in the extraction process is selecting the desired flowers, herbs, or roots you want to extract into oil form. This can be done either through harvesting your own plants, buying them from stores that sell fresh plant material, or ordering them online from other providers. Once you have finished your selection, it will need to be dried thoroughly in order for the oils inside the plant material to develop properly and not spoil once they have been extracted. This is accomplished by wrapping the plant material in cheesecloth, placing it in a drying oven, or simply placing it on a windowsill. When the drying process is finished, you can move on to the next step of your extraction.

The next step is placing the dried plant material into an oil press or using other equipment that involves pressing liquid to extract the oils from their raw form into an oil form. This can be accomplished by using a simple device called an "oil press" or purchasing one for specific purposes, an activated charcoal press, and a winepress. Also, if you are making sugar alcohol extractions, then using a water-free alcohol press (also referred to as a reverse osmosis system) is sufficient.

After the oil press has extracted the oil, it is then heated and distilled through steam to remove unwanted contents of the oil. This process removes dirt and other particulates from the final product. After this, the oil can be bottled and labeled for use.

The first step in essential oils is to find a starting material, and in this case, we will be using flowers, herbs, or roots. The first step in greasing a plant material is usually drying it out; if it's green, then drying it out will make sure that your final product doesn't spoil easily. A drying oven or other means of heat is used to do this.

Once the plant material has been dried out and placed into a jar, it will need to be macerated, which means that you are pulverizing the flowers, herbs, or roots in a mortar and pestle until they are thick paste. First, you want to get rid of any large chunks that are stuck in the plant materials. You can do this by grinding them with your pestle until their separation occurs.

Next, you need to combine the liquid with a non-polar solvent, such as alcohol or water. This allows for better mixing up of the material and less chance of contamination. All that is left is adding carrier oil, like olive oil if desired—storing your final solution—and then moving on to the extraction!

The first step in extraction is removing any solvents or impurities from your starting material by macerating it with a solvent such as water (if using an oil press) or alcohol (if using an alcohol press). This will make the solvent penetrate in and dissolve the plant material in order to get it ready for extraction. After the maceration, you can use an oil press instead of an alcohol press instead of an oil press, whichever is preferred.

After the macerating and extraction, the oils will need to be dried out to prevent spoilage. Dryers are used to accomplish this step, and the process is similar to maceration, with a few differences. To begin, dryers allow for airflow around the oil rather than substance; this is accomplished by drying it in a warm room, such as the attic or sunroom, or using a dehydrator. Drying out the oil will take time, so this is the best time to write up labels and make sure that you are containing the oil properly.

With almost all extracts, you will want to clean out your equipment after use. After this process, it is always best to let the equipment dry for a few extra days so that there is no chance of mold growth or other possible contaminants.

When making essential oils with fresh plant material, you will need to leave a lot of space for the final product because they have a tendency to expand quite a lot during extraction and drying. The following are the labels that will ensure that the oil is stored properly:

The most common method of extraction in essential oils is to use an oil press, which stands for "oil press" and is also known as a cold press or "activated charcoal press." The process of using an oil press to make essential oils is similar to other distilled products.

Another popular method of extraction involves using alcohol instead of water. For this method, you need to create a solution with water and alcohol. The following are the labels that will ensure that the alcohol has been properly treated. A popular method of extraction involves using alcohol. This can be done either by mixing water and alcohol or by mixing them separately and then combining them with the plant material, much like a water-based extraction.

If you manufacture sugar alcohol extracts, such as those containing sorbitol or mannitol, then you will want to use an airless extraction machine. This machine allows for the sugar alcohol to be processed and extracted into a solution. If you are making sugar alcohol extracts, then you will want to use an airless extraction machine. Many of the benefits of this machine are that it can be used with plants as well as fruits and candy, both of which are good sources for sugar alcohol extract. The device is used in order to extract the sugars from the plant material.

After the processing is complete, you should heat up all of your equipment to 130°F in order to make sure that there are no risks of contaminants or unwanted processes after your product has been extracted and dried out.

Many people who make essential oils experience difficulty in finding a good way to store the oils. It is important that you have proper storage methods in place to make sure that your essential oil products do not expire quickly. Maintaining the proper conditions will allow your product to have a longer shelf life and also help prevent contamination. Storage methods are made up of several ways, which should be used for containers with airtight lids, so you can be sure that your product will not spoil before it is needed.

All types of essential oil storage should include cold, dry, dark space; no sunlight or light exposure; no direct heat source (heat-based diffusers, ovens, etc.); temperature above 68 degrees; no exposure to water or spray.

Both aromatherapy and flower essences are based on the theory that when you inhale or ingest certain fragrances, they can affect your emotional state. Flower essences are made from flowers, leaves, bark, roots, and fruits. They're diluted in water to create a tea-like drink. Aromatherapy is the practice of using various aromatic substances to improve one's mood or physical condition.

Aromatherapy has been used for many centuries as a healing process — both physically and mentally — while it has only been recently that flower essences have gained popularity in the west. The aroma of a real flower can be compared to 50–70 chemicals in one. These chemicals vary greatly by species, and for this reason, it is difficult to compare one essence with another. Therefore, we should look at how flower essences are created and the results they produce when used.

In order for the essence to gain your attention, it must have a positive image or metaphor that will entice you, as a perfume would do. The analogy that I like to use in regard to this is that of "seduced by smell" as opposed to "seduced by vision." Flowers are not only aromatic plants that get us high, but they are also very beautiful and intricate. A collection of plants can be likened to a flower shop surrounded by fragrant, colorful blooms.

This analogy does a good job of demonstrating the differences between the effects produced by essence and that of a real flower. An essence smells good because it is made up of molecules that resemble those in the natural world. In contrast, when you inhale the smell of flowers (real or artificial), they have no effect on our nervous system because it isn't necessary for survival, as flowers don't produce food and thus aren't necessary for survival, whereas essential oils are needed for this.

How to Prepare Essential Oils

Essential oils are liquid extracts of a variety of plants that have the potential to be useful. The valuable chemicals from these plants can be extracted using manufacturing procedures. Essential oils have a stronger scent and contain more active chemicals than the plants they are derived from. This is due to the amount of plant matter needed to produce essential oil.

Solvent Extraction

The chemical components of most flowers are too gentle to destroy nature by the high heat used in steam distillation, yet they contain too slight volatile oil to be expressed. So instead, the oils are extracted using a solvent such as supercritical, hexane, or CO2.

Concretes are a blend of essential herbal oil, resins, waxes, and other oil-soluble (lipophilic) plants substantially extracted from hexane and hydrophobic solvents. Concretes include a lot of non-aromatic resins and waxes, although they're quite fragrant.

The fragrant oil is frequently extracted from the concrete using another solvent, such as ethyl alcohol. The waxes and lipids precipitate after the alcohol solution is refrigerated to 18°C (0°F) for more than 48 hours. The precipitates are then filtered out, and the ethanol in the remaining solution is detached by vacuum purge, evaporation, or both, leaving the absolute.

In the extraction of supercritical fluids, supercritical carbon dioxide is often used as a solvent. This process avoids petrochemical residues in the product and the loss of some "top notes compared to steam distillation." However, it doesn't directly produce an absolute. Both the essential oils and waxes in the concrete will be extracted using supercritical carbon dioxide.

Separating the waxes from the essential oils requires additional processing with liquefied carbon dioxide, which can be accomplished in the same extractor by reducing the extraction temperature. Compounds do not decompose or denaturize as a result of this lower temperature procedure. When the extraction is finished, the pressure is dropped to ambient, and the carbon dioxide turns back into a gas, leaving no residue.

Obtaining Florasols

Another solvent for extracting essential oils is "Floral 134a." It was created as a substitute for "Freon" as a refrigerant. Floral has a high global warming potential (GWP; 100-year GWP = 1430), despite being an "ozone-friendly" substance. As a result, the European Union has outlawed its use, with a phase-out period starting in 2011 and ending in 2017.

Floral has the advantage of extracting essential oils at or below room temperature, which prevents degradation due to high temperatures.

How Do Essential Oils Work?

Aromatherapy, in which essential oils are breathed through various techniques, is the most prevalent use of essential oils. Essential oils never are consumed. They include molecules or particles that interrelate with the body in different ways.

Some plant composites are absorbed when applied to the skin. Some application methods, such as applying with heat or to various parts of the body, are thought to rise absorption. However, research is scarce in this field.

Essential oil fragrances can trigger portions of your brain, or more precisely, the limbic system, which is involved in behaviors, scent, emotions, and long-term memory.

Unexpectedly, the limbic system plays a major role in the formation of memory. Therefore, it may help in clarifying why certain smells might elicit emotions or memories.

The brain's limbic system also controls several involuntary physiological activities, including blood, respiration, and heart rate, and pressure. Therefore, it is assumed that essential oils have a physical impact on the human body. Essential oils can be inhaled or applied to the skin after being diluted. When ingested, they may heighten your sense of smell or have medical properties.

Essential Oils Used by Native Americans

An intense hydrophobic liquid holding volatile chemical components from plants is known as an "essential oil." Volatile oils, petroleum, and ethereal oils (or simply the plant-soil from which they were extracted by flowers, roots, leaves, wood, bars, seed, or peel) are used to describe essential oils. Essential oils are "essential" in the manner that they have the "essence of" the plant's scent, which is the distinctive scent of the herb or plant from which it was extracted.

Aromatherapy was employed in ancient ceremonies to combat pessimism and evil. According to our forefathers, good scents fend off evil spirits and keep wicked creatures at a distance. The herbal oils were employed to get rid of bad items for people's health and well-being. Aromatherapy, strongly argued, has a major effect on one's life and should be required in all types of emotional, physical, spiritual, or psychological purification. It was recommended by everyone from the prehistoric Egyptians to the Romans, Greeks, Persians, and Hindus as an alternative type of medicine.

History of Essential Oils

Throughout history, essential oils have been employed in traditional medicine. The Persian surgeon Ibn Sina, acknowledged in Europe as Avicenna, was the first to originate the Attar or scent of flowers from the distillation method, while Ibn al-Baitar, who was an Arabic-Spanish Muslim general practitioner, chemist, and pharmacist, is thought to be the first to mention the techniques and methods used to produce essential oils.

Rather than referring to essential oils as a whole, current publications frequently mention single chemical compounds that make up essential oils, such as "methyl salicylate" instead of "wintergreen oil." Aromatherapy has reignited interest in herbal essential oils in recent decades. Volatilized oils are utilized in massage, disseminated in the atmosphere with a nebulizer or diffuser (burned as incense), and a candle flame was used to heat it.

Native Americans and their Aromatherapy

The herbal oils have long been used by Native Americans and ancient civilizations in their everyday routines and spiritual and domestic rituals.

They have a deep admiration for Mother Nature and utilize only natural products in their daily lives. They think that the herbal oils, with their potent scents, may ward off evil spirits while also improving their overall health. For example, aromatic oils and herbs are used in Native American cleaning rituals. Aromatic herbs such as sage, sweet grass, cedar wood, juniper, pine spikes, and others help in purifying and ridding the air of bad energies to appeal positivity into life. But why would we discuss aromatherapy in the Native American tradition? It is simple, practical, primal, and very natural.

Americans have a broader understanding of aromatherapy than other aromatherapists do, and they recognize which oils or plants can be used to combat strong emotions, mental turmoil, and other negative energy in life. The majority of the Natives' herbs and oils are widely available and obtained at aromatherapy shops and online stores. They employ herbs in their most pure and natural state as aromatic plants with fragrances rather than making appealing combinations (as many aromatherapists do).

Smudging Is a Native American Ritual

Smudging is a sacred American Indian tradition that entails burning plants for purification and prayer, and the vast majority of American Indians practice it.

In addition, the burning of the herbs unleashes various pleasant scents from the plant's oils, which adds to the whole experience. The herbs' smoke is then used to offer prayers.

Smudging is a spiritual healing ritual that may include people passing burning herbs from one person to the next in communal prayer to the Creator. Sweet grass and sage are two common smudging plants. Bergamot, yarrow, mesquite, bearberry, and tobacco are other herbs used for smudging alone or in mixes.

The smoke from the burning of sage and sweet grass is thought to carry prayers and sorrows up to the spirits in spiritual rites. Medical applications offered by individuals selling medicinal oils range from skincare treatment to cancer treatments, and they are frequently based simply on historical records of essential oil use for these purposes. In most countries, claims about the efficacy of medical therapies, particularly cancer therapy, are now regulated.

Part VII

~

Herbal Remedies

Introduction

 A Native American herbal remedy is an ancient indigenous remedy that has been made from the plants and other materials used by native North Americans. They are usually made by water extraction, without the use of modern machinery or chemicals. While some herbs have been harvested for thousands of years, others are still being slowly gathered in their natural habitats.

Native American herbs were primarily used as remedies for different problems, such as physical maladies or spiritual conditions such as depression. The effectiveness of these remedies is also attributable to their ritual use, which can often increase their healing potential. Since they do not include any harmful ingredients, like some over-the-counter drugs, they have a lower risk for side effects than most pharmaceuticals do.

Many Native Americans have used a vast variety of tribal herbs to treat various ailments and heal themselves. Many of these people have used the knowledge passed to them by their ancestors to come up with natural remedies for one thing or another, and in some cases, they have combined plant parts to make medicines for multiple conditions. Some Native Americans (most notably the Cherokee) have even used herbs in place of surgery.

The Cherokee rosehip was one popular ingredient that was used in many preparations. The Cherokee would often use this part of the plant either in an infusion or tincture form for both internal and external treatment purposes. Many other common herbs used by Native American tribes have also been used for medicinal purposes, in addition to being used for ritual purposes.

The plants that were being used by native people had many valuable properties. One frequently mentioned herb was the native tobacco plant, which has several various alkaloids within its many parts. Because of this, they have been used as a remedy for irritable bowel syndrome and cancers. Other herbs such as willow bark were often taken in tea form in order to help with colds and sore throats.

Many plants are used in Native American herbal remedies. Some of the herbs include the American ginseng, all parts of the sassafras tree, marshmallow root, and poke sallet root. There are also various other types of plants that were used, including goldenrod, copperhead weed root, black haw bark, dandelion herb, and many others. Some cultures use different forms of these herbs, such as the Abnaki Indians, in which they use either crushed roots or root bark in order to treat hypertension and coughs.

The Cherokee herbalists have also used the elderberry leaf for a variety of ailments, including heart palpitations, occasional fainting spells, as well as the prevention of influenza and colds. Numerous other herbs are used in Native American herbal remedies, such as the white oak acorns. These acorns were often mixed with various plants in order to treat skin complaints, wounds, and even infections.

The tribes that didn't have access to the much-needed medical knowledge or treatments often had medicine men that would try to provide treatments using whatever they had available at their disposal. This ranged from tobacco leaves to the roots of plants. While the techniques used by the medicine men varied in accordance with the different tribes, their medicinal knowledge, and herbal remedies were much more widespread than modern medicine.

A Brief Overview

Native Americans have been using herbs for beauty, health, and general well-being for centuries. They have never had a formalized system of medicine as it is recognized by the health care industry today. Rather, they relied on hundreds of plants to treat a wide variety of ailments.

A Brief History of Native American Medicine

There is evidence of Native Americans healing each other from at least 1800 BCE. Evidence suggests that many healers used whole plant remedies, as well as some animal parts. However, there is also a history of catching and drying herbs for use in the future. Many treatments utilized little or no processing.

Native Americans treated diseases differently than European settlers did, and these treatments followed different principles than we do today. One consequence was that it became difficult to establish a standard of care among groups, making it difficult for doctors who came to live with the tribe and treat its members. This resulted in short-term solutions being used to address long-term problems—sometimes with disastrous results. Another problem was that medicines were not tested consistently to ensure safety; therefore, many Native American remedies still contain unknown and possibly dangerous chemicals.

What Is Native American Herbal Medicine?

Native American herbal medicine includes the use of plants, such as sagebrush, cattails, and elderberries, for health and beauty.

There are a variety of different types of Native American herbal remedies: treating colds with willow branches; applying a paste on the chest to treat rheumatic pain; using bear's milk as a shampoo to heal scalps and making extracts from the roots of plants to alleviate joint pain.

Chamomile is a popular natural remedy used to treat digestive problems, but some European settlers thought it was harmful. Some believed it was a gonorrhea treatment (a venereal disease), while others thought it caused leprosy in children. The confusion ended when Dr. H.E Hooker, a botanist, confirmed that Native Americans were using chamomile correctly.

Medicine men are considered the most important herbalists in Native American culture because of their extensive knowledge and history of healing. Medicine men often specialize in one area, such as treating colds or providing pain relief for women during childbirth.

Native Americans have also used different herbs to change their physical appearance. Some individuals used a mixture of different herbs to lighten their skin, while others used a concoction of berries to dye their hair red.

Historically, the Native American population has suffered from a lack of access to quality health care and an inability to afford the cost of that care when it is available. Some tribes offer free clinics through their tribal affiliation, but this is not always the case. This is compounded by a general distrust expressed by many Native Americans towards strangers in white coats and towards certain aspects of mainstream medicine.

The cost of health care insurance is also of concern to many Native Americans and a focus of many discussions. Most tribal health care funding comes from the federal government, which can be inconsistent and unpredictable.

There is an expression among those who have worked with Native Americans: "You can't make a good person healthy." This belief advocate that—regardless of how effective our treatments are—we will never be successful unless we first focus on the holistic healing of the entire person. Only then can we hope to help people reclaim their culture, identity, self-worth, and ultimately their health. Only then will we be successful in achieving our core mission as herbalists: "The restoration to health by the use of plants."

Native American herbal remedies are essential to the preservation of Native American culture. They have been used for centuries in ceremonies and rituals to help bless and cleanse people before they enter a sacred space. In modern times, they continue to be used as treatments for a wide range of ailments. For example, green tea is often used by warriors in ceremonies because it helps relieve stress and boosts energy levels.

Common Problems

Herbal Remedies Side Effects

If you've ever considered taking herbal remedies for your health, be aware that they can have serious side effects.

How do you know if the herbs will cause a negative reaction to other treatments? Herbal remedies are not well-regulated and tests have not been conducted to find out how they may interact with prescription medicines.

The dangers of herbal medicine include interacting with other medicines, high drug and herb concentrations, unlisted ingredients, or contaminants from natural sources. An unknown ingredient could lead to an allergic reaction or other unforeseen complications. Contaminated herbs or bacterial or fungal contamination in plants can cause serious health problems.

If you do not have a doctor's prescription for herbal remedies, it is important that you watch out for the following conditions:

An overdose could result in dizziness, blurred vision, dilated pupils, slurred speech, and raised body temperature. The most common side effect of taking herbal remedies is nausea, but some can also cause skin rashes and allergic reactions such as hives.

Always check labels carefully before taking any herbal remedy. Herbal remedies which are thought to be "all-natural" are not always safe, and no testing has ever been done to find out how they might interact with prescription medicine or other supplements.

Before taking any herbal medicine, it is important that you be sure to read the following:

- If you are taking a blood thinner such as warfarin, ask your doctor what would happen when you take these remedies. It may be possible that they will interact and cause dangerously low blood pressure (hypotension) or bleeding in the event of injury, surgery, or dentistry. Some medications can interfere with herbs and cause serious side effects. Do not take herbal remedies if you are pregnant or breastfeeding.

- Many herbal remedies have harmful interactions when taken with certain foods and herbs. This is due to "herb-drug" interactions, in which a supplement can interfere with a medication your body is currently taking. However, other substances such, as milk or alcohol, can also cause issues for some medications.

- Since herbal remedies have not been well studied, it can be difficult to know what interactions might occur if they are taken in combination with certain medications or supplements. Therefore, doctors do not necessarily know what interactions will occur when a particular herbal remedy is combined with other agents. Doctors recommend that patients unfamiliar with herbs read all product labels and ask their doctor's advice on the safe use of herbal remedies in combination with prescription medicines.

This is because herbal remedies often contain a variety of ingredients that can be present in varying amounts. Therefore, it's important to use herbs that are approved by FDA and meet GMP regulations.

Herbal remedies are not well-regulated and tests have not been conducted to find out how they may interact with prescription medicines.

To understand herbal remedies meaning, you will have to check the composition of the herbal remedy by yourself. Be aware of any drug interactions caused by the herbal remedies. Herbal remedies can also cause serious side effects if taken with other drugs or foods. While they have been around for thousands of years, it is important to remember that herbs are not drugs and not all herbs are safe in all situations.

Disadvantages of Using Herbal Remedies

There are many types of herbal remedies available today. Numerous people choose to use these herbal remedies in place of traditional medications. This is because they believe that the medicines they are taking are more beneficial to their health than the medications prescribed by a doctor, and can help relieve certain medical conditions without potential side effects from traditional medicine. However, there are some disadvantages to using herbal remedies which many people might not be aware of.

There is not much scientific evidence to support the effectiveness of herbal remedies. Some people who use these natural methods of treatment may believe that they are effective, but there are no valid clinical studies to prove it. Even if studies did exist, the results would most likely be very limited since so many herbal remedies are available. This leaves doctors and scientists with very little data to help them make educated decisions.

Herbal remedies can contain dangerous chemicals and/or contaminants. Many people erroneously believe that all herbs are natural products and therefore safe to use. However, this may not always be true, since some mushrooms in the world have harmful toxins in them which can cause severe damage. Herbal remedies imported from other countries may contain chemicals and contaminants which are dangerous because they have never been tested. Herbs grown in areas with polluted air or water may contain harmful contaminants such as heavy metals and pesticides, which could be potentially harmful to humans.

Herbal remedies do not always work well with traditional medications. Many times, people take herbal remedies when they are also taking other medications without consulting their doctor first, which can result in serious side effects or failure in their treatment. If you are taking any medications for your health problems, you should always consult your doctor about the herbal remedies you would like to take so that he or she can advise you on whether these natural treatments will work well with your current medical treatments or not.

Herbal remedies are not required to be tested or approved by the FDA, which means that there is no assurance that they actually contain what they claim to contain. There have been numerous cases where ingredients have been added into herbal remedies without the knowledge of the manufacturers or distributors, which could decrease their effectiveness.

Herbal remedies can leave you with toxic build-up if you continue to use them too frequently. Some people believe that taking a dose of herbs on a daily basis will make them immune to these illnesses and diseases naturally, but this is far from true. Herbs used for the treatment of a particular disease or ailment should be taken on an as-needed basis. This means that you should only take them when you are suffering from symptoms of a particular illness or ailment, and not on a daily or even weekly basis.

There is no regulation to measure the potency of herbal remedies for most herbs, which may be due to their being considered a natural substance. The lack of regulation can also cause manufacturing errors in supplements which can have harmful effects if they contain excessive amounts of ingredients like herbs and oils which have been diluted to make the herb look more potent (which may not always be the case).

Many people take herbal remedies when they are suffering from a disease or ailment, but no evidence proves that herbal remedies can treat any specific disease and/or ailment. This means that there is no scientific data to prove the safety and effectiveness of many of these products.

Herbal remedies may be mislabeled by manufacturers. This may occur when an ingredient in an herbal remedy has been intentionally altered by the manufacturer without your knowledge; this could result in serious health problems for you if you take these supplements regularly.

Many herbal remedies contain ingredients that have negative side effects. Many people believe that herbal remedies are completely safe to use, but this is not always the case. Certain ingredients found in specific herbal remedies may cause harmful side effects if you take them on a regular basis, or if you take high amounts of these supplements.

Herbs and essential oils used in the preparation of certain herbal remedies may contain alcohol, which could have negative side effects for your health if you consume a large enough amount of it.

How Herbs Work

Herbs are commonly used for medicinal purposes. However, not all herbs work in the same way and usually have more than one effect. Paprika is used widely as a spice and as a treatment for certain skin conditions, but it has been scientifically proven to prevent some types of cancer cells from growing. However, fresh paprika should not be used to treat cancer because it lacks the necessary nutrients needed for healing purposes in large doses.

Benefits of Growing Medicinal Plants

The benefits of medicinal plant gardening are many and varied. Not only does it provide an opportunity to connect deeply with nature, but it also provides the opportunity to grow your own pharmaceutical that would otherwise be too expensive. Medicinal plants are best utilized in natural remedies because they can often contain valuable ingredients such as menthol, camphor, carvacrol, thymol, eugenol, citronellal, and more.

Doctors have been prescribing medicinal plants for centuries before they eventually synthesized them into drugs. Medicinal plants were the first source of drugs that antibiotics derived from mold fungi centuries later, for example! Aside from the obvious health benefits, growing your own medicinal plants also gives you a chance to grow rare or uncommon species that you may not have access to otherwise.

Many ingredients found in medicinal plants are known for their anti-bacterial, anti-fungal, analgesic, and anti-inflammatory properties. These types of beneficial ingredients can help treat many common ailments, such as acne, burns, earaches, colds, and more. Growing your own medicinal plants is one way of ensuring you always have a supply on hand to use when needed.

Medicinal plant gardening is an ideal way to learn about natural remedies too. Many plants you grow, if they are left to flower, will attract pollinating insects and butterflies and can even help control pests.

If you're looking to improve your health, reduce pain or get yourself back on track with your nutrition and diet, medicinal plants may just be the answer for you. You can grow them in containers so that they are easily transported around your home as needed too.

Medicinal plants are also excellent if you're looking to de-stress and relax. The helpful nature of medicinal plants can help you tackle your daily stress positively. They can also be used to help improve your mood and energy levels. It is also very relaxing to grow your medicinal plants in your own garden and many of the common ingredients found in them will naturally help you sleep better at night.

It can be very rewarding to grow or even learn about medicinal plants, as they can provide many useful benefits. The best part about growing your own medicinal plants; however, is the fact that you have a chance to learn something new or fine-tune, an old remedy that you've been using for years. It can be very rewarding too as you'll be able to stop relying on prescription medications one day soon too! Medicinal plant gardening is easy and rewarding.

You don't even have to be an expert gardener to start growing medicinal plants. It is best if you know a little bit about growing plants before you get started, though.

Conditions Treated by Native American Medicine

Eating disorders, such as anorexia and bulimia, are fast becoming a prevalent problem in our society. Many with these conditions lack the skills to set boundaries and to stand up for them. Others suffer from low self-esteem. The list of conditions treated by Native American Medicine is extensive, but in this article, I will focus on those which are particularly relevant to young women such as eating disorders as well as depression and anxiety.

In Native American medicine, we do not view these diseases as a disease in the conventional sense, but rather we treat their underlying causes. The causes of eating disorders can be emotional or spiritual, often rooted in the misunderstanding of a child's spiritual identity and purpose; sometimes they are a symptom of excess energy that needs to be transformed into something positive or they may simply be a cry for help from someone who feels lost and alone.

Native American Medicine does not view eating disorders as being a disease in the way we do. We consider eating disorders as being an imbalance caused by an emotional, spiritual or mental issue and nothing more. This is why Native American Medicine treats every individual according to their unique situation and condition. The causes of these conditions range from the simple to the complex. Some causes are clearly visible on a physical level; others can be seen in the form of rashes, bloating, stomach cramps, headaches, or other physical symptoms that can easily become confused with other diagnoses like food poisoning or an infection

Native American Medicine is not only limited to the treatment of eating disorders, but also can be used to help with other conditions such as "burnout" (which is a term coined by Dr. Jordan Peterson), grief, stress, and self-esteem issues. If you or someone you know suffers from an eating disorder or another specific condition, I strongly recommend you seek a shamanic consultation. A shamanic consultation can assist in getting to the root of the problem and assisting in healing. A shamanic consultation may be helpful if you are seeking a way out of the "disease," as some physical symptoms will disappear once you have set free yourself from the emotional cause that was behind it all along.

In my practice, I help people come to understand their spirituality and purpose in the world. Once you understand why you are on this earth, so many of these physical "diseases" will disappear. If an eating disorder arises because a person has a strong need to protect herself from the world once that has been dealt with, then the eating disorder will no longer be necessary. This is why Native American Medicine does not treat disease but rather works with the person to heal what ails them and assist them in living a healthier balanced life.

Today I will be using an example of a client that came to me with symptoms of bloating, nausea, and headaches. When I asked her about her life, she told me she was very stressed with school. I noticed that she was taking care of others to the point that they were becoming her priority and not herself. She had let herself go, even though she was very young for a woman of her age.

As we talked more, it became apparent that she had deeply buried emotions regarding past trauma. Some were so deep and buried and others were so recent that they had not yet been addressed or processed on an emotional level.

I recommend that you read this part from the shamanic perspective. I want to be clear; Native American Medicine does not view trancework as a solution for all problems, and certainly not in every case. In this article, I am just using an example of how to work with someone who is experiencing symptoms of anxiety or low self-esteem. If you are suffering from an eating disorder, please seek help from a professional. This is about creating healthy boundaries and seeing yourself as an important part of the world around you.

When we work with someone using Native American Medicine, we can choose to work on an emotional level or a spiritual level. It is important to note that what I mean by "spiritual" here is not necessarily in the religious sense; it is more about the way you view yourself and your purpose in life.

The way you treat yourself can have a big impact on how others treat you as well. When we work with people who have eating disorders, the symptoms may include bloating, stomachaches, and headaches. I have even seen cases where a person has lost consciousness from experiencing symptoms like these.

Some people are very afraid of going to hospitals or seeing doctors because they don't know how to explain what they are feeling or experiencing. If you are suffering from any of these symptoms, it is important to seek professional help.

What I hope you take away from this article is that a shamanic consultation can be very helpful in helping get to the root of what is happening. If an eating disorder arises for any reason, it's important to seek out professional help.

After the consultation, you may find that you are so relieved that it will be easy to make healthy choices for yourself and live a normal life again. I have helped many people come to a place of self-love and peace. When this happens, their body starts to heal itself and they stop making unhealthy lifestyle choices. This is why Native American Medicine can be considered a "disease cure" or "anti-disease vaccine."

In traditional Native American medicine, there were six healing practices: the sweat lodge, the tea ceremony, herbal remedies, massage therapy, fasting, and abstinence from certain foods and behaviors. Traditional healers were not limited to the treatment of physical ailments; they also treated mental disorders like depression. A common belief that Western Medicine is superior to Native American medicine is false. The treatments used by Native Americans have been proven to be effective. Native American medicine is effective because it has been passed down by generations of healers who have used the knowledge for centuries. Source: National Museum of the American Indian.

Native American Medicine is distinct from medical systems found among other Amerindian groups. The healing practices amongst many Native tribes, like that of the Apache and Lakota Sioux, are based on an understanding of spiritual and ecological realities rather than modern scientific understanding.

Throughout the United States, there are hundreds of thousands of people who practice traditional native medicine to some degree. The people who practice this system believe in a holistic approach to health and healing.

Indian doctors believed that physical, mental, and spiritual health were inseparable components of our beings, which depended on the balance of two forces in nature: light and dark. This concept was described as "two-into-one" medicine. It was believed that illness originated when one force was out of balance. Certain traditional practices were used to restore balance, and to treat illness, including prayer, sweat lodges, and herbal remedies. These practices were also used to strengthen the immune system, and to keep diseases of the body in check. The Native American doctor also believed that illness resulted from an imbalance of emotions.

There were five means of re-establishing health and healing:

- "Holy men who healed through prayer."
- The sweat-lodge ceremony.
- "Medicine Songs," chants that were sung over drums or flutes, treated physical ailments as well as emotional disorders by singing.
- "Wilderness fasting."
- "Herbal remedies and teas."

Native American doctors used the following herbs for healing:

- Sage.
- Catnip.
- Valerian.
- Yarrow.
- Stinging nettle.
- Mullein leaves.
- Hawthorn leaves.

The most common Native American medical practices involved herbal remedies. The plant most widely used was sage, which Native Americans used for a variety of illnesses and diseases, including snake bites, colds, coughs, and sore throats.

To treat diseases and physical pain, Native American doctors used poultices—ointments that were applied to the skin. Poultices were made up of a wide variety of herbs, including yarrow, which was thought to be good for treating wounds. Another poultice was made up of the inner bark of trees, such as mullein and laurel. This bark was an arthritis treatment, fever, and skin disease. Another poultice was made from the roots of black cherry bushes.

This poultice was used to treat boils, sores, and infections in wounds.

Native American medicine has some similarities to Western medicine, but there are many differences. One of the biggest differences between these two systems is the way they are administered. In Native American healing, certain herbs are used to treat illnesses and diseases in the body. Herbal remedies and teas are also given to treat psychological disorders.

The Spirit of Healing

For The Spirit of Healing, everything begins with the human spirit. The Spirit of Healing experience is a living embodiment of the healing energy that we believe to be present in each person.

The spirit of healing values is based on this belief. We believe that every person has the potential to heal themselves and others. Everyone has something positive to offer, and it's up to everyone to find their own unique way of sharing that gift.

The Spirit of Healing experience centers on our commitment to a holistic approach to health and well-being. We recognize that a harmonious relationship with our bodies, minds, and spirits is the only truly effective path toward optimal health and fitness.

Our holistic approach means that we support many forms of alternative medicine. Many people choose to incorporate Native American traditions into their healing practices, meditation, prayer, and more.

At the spirit of healing, we believe that everyone can benefit from all forms of healing, including traditional Western medicine, naturopathic care, herbal medicine, acupuncture, homeopathic remedies, massage therapy, yoga classes, and physical therapy. We recognize that no one path is better than another in terms of healing power. All paths have merit when used together in order to create a healthy lifestyle.

"Spirit" means to have a deep connection with a thing. A connection that allows for healing, comfort, and growth. If you've ever seen your pet or child, or anyone that you love, grow from seed to seed, you know how powerful the word "spirit" can be.

The concept behind the Spirit of Healing is simple: We offer an alternative to health insurance and medical providers in the event that medical emergencies arise. We believe in the power of healing and we want to help you and your family stay healthy and safe when you need it most.

When you're not feeling well, it's hard to think clearly. You might not be able to call a health care provider at the time of injury or illness, or you might delay seeking treatment for fear of high costs or inability to pay. Our way of treating injuries and illnesses is designed to empower families to take action quickly when they need it most.

The Spirit of Healing is an ancient Native American tradition. The roots of this spiritual tradition have existed for thousands of years and are still being practiced today.

Many people believe that Native American spirits are categorized as good or bad, but this is not accurate. The Spirit of Healing is a spiritual energy that protects all living things from harm. If you are in need of help, seek out a medicine person or spiritual healer and ask to be healed. This can be done by kissing the ground, offering a prayer, or even having an item touching your body in a prescribed manner. While various Indian tribes may approach the healing process in different ways, the underlying concept is universal. The Spirit of Healing is a universal energy that everyone possesses and that all people can access on a daily basis.

This energy can be tapped into by anyone who decides to do so, whether they are a shaman, a healer, or an artist. When I first learned how to access and work with this energy, I was instantly captivated. It is a beautiful and powerful gift that is available to all of us.

The power of the spirit is accessed through the breath. When you slow down your breathing and breathe deeply, you are allowing yourself to open up and allow the spirit to flow into your body. Through this process, you begin to access the power within you and channel it into your healing work.

When I first began working with the spirit, I was amazed at how easy it became part of my daily life. Although I didn't understand it at first, I soon realized that it had an amazing way of helping me through the challenges of my life and providing solutions to problems that were out of my control.

I began by using the breath as a means of releasing tension in my muscles at night before going to bed. Through this nightly ritual, I was able to reset myself for the day and begin each day with a clear mind and an open heart. This simple change had a profound effect on my life. Soon I realized that it helped when I was working on artwork as well.

I had been practicing meditation for years before learning about the spirit's power in therapy sessions with patients who were dealing with anxiety disorders or other problems caused by their daily struggles in life. Within hours, after setting up a meditation ritual in their homes, they would notice an immediate improvement in their mental well-being, which would continue for the rest of their lives.

Part VIII

~

A Natural Approach to Common Aliments

Aging

Aging is a natural process that happens to everyone. It is important to be proactive about aging, and take care of your body and skin as best as possible! This chapter will list some anti-aging tea recipes and their benefits.

The process of aging is a controlled process by the body, which is important to consider as we age. The rate at which we age is controlled by two factors: metabolism and genes. As people age, their metabolism begins to slow down and cells are not able to produce energy as efficiently as they did when they were younger. The body has a natural repair rate (which is why your skin does not regenerate) but the rate at which it repairs itself slows down with age.

Growing is an inevitable part of life. As people experience growth, their age, and with aging, there are various and drastic changes in terms of physical and even emotional aspects. However, they can be treated or prevented through different herbal medicines. Technically, aging is the natural change that could normally occur in early adulthood. More than the physical changes, one's body function deteriorates as well. Thus, people have different aging patterns; it is typically the same as the era that they experienced it. They might also experience different and unique symptoms, but it all boils down to aging. Historically, aging starts at the age of sixty-five; however, it was based on the required retirement age.

Biologically, there is no exact age for it. The known symptoms of aging are thickening of the eye's lens, stiffens, and presbyopia.

Curcumin

It is known to have an anti-aging property due to its compounds. It is also listed to have a compound like turmeric, which implies another property like antioxidant, a known property for brightening the skin. Moreover, it is also tagged to be a fighter against cellular damage. Having this benefit could postpone diseases that are triggered with age. Turmeric is a great alternative for curcumin.

In most recipes, turmeric is used as an alternative for curcumin, just like for its skin polisher and moisturizing mask. For the skin polisher, the ingredients needed are one tablespoon of gram flour, one-fourth teaspoon of turmeric, and two teaspoons of milk. The ingredients are only needed to be mixed. Afterward, they can be directly used for the skin. It must be rubbed, left on for ten minutes, and can be washed off with the fingers. The water must be specifically warm. On the other hand, turmeric can be added to honey to create a moisturizing mask. The things needed are one tablespoon of organic honey and a teaspoon of turmeric. Like the polisher, they are only needed to be mixed and be applied. However, the mask needs a longer time of setting; it must be sitting on the face for fifteen to twenty minutes. And for its rising, it also needs lukewarm water.

Basil

It is important in preventing the symptoms. Aging could be triggered by too much exposure to UV light; it could damage the skin and it could cause depletion of the collagens.

Collagen is identified to be the reason why the skin is able to be elastic for a long time. Once it breaks down, the quality of the skin deteriorates. Basil could help in maintaining the quality of the skin by moisturizing it. It can stop the roughness of the skin, same with its scaliness. It could also prevent the skin to attain wrinkles. Its only goal is to make the skin beautiful and smooth.

To be able to use basil as an anti-aging medicine, it should be mixed with a tablespoon of gram flour and a teaspoon of honey. The basil leaves must be exactly a cup. First, the basil leaves have to be boiled in warm water until it produces a paste-like texture. When the texture is achieved, the gram flour and the honey are needed to be mixed.

When they are well-mixed already, the finished product is also ready for application. When applied, let it sit until it gets dry. Afterward, rinse it off with lukewarm water.

Asthma

Asthma is a chronic disease affecting the airways. It leads to a narrowing of the airways, which can then restrict breathing. Asthma causes attacks characterized by airflow obstruction (recurrent bronchospasm), wheezing, chest tightness, and coughing.

Individuals with asthma usually have increased sensitivity in both their lungs and the muscles around them that help people breathe (bronchi). The increased sensitivity means that these individuals will respond strongly to triggers like allergens, cold weather/dry air/exercise. This is why, for many people with asthma, an asthma attack may be triggered by talking or laughing too hard or by going outside on a cold day without warm clothes. Individuals with asthma have increased reactivity of these muscles, which leads to narrowing of the airways. Bronchospasm is the name given to muscle contraction (the narrowing of the airways). As a result, during an asthma attack, air can only pass through the narrowed pathway, making it harder to breathe.

Natural Treatment Treatments Cure Asthma

You already realize that pharmaceutical medications are the greatest medication expense linked to asthma, whether you have asthma or concern about someone who does. Asthma treatment in the United States costs $6 billion a year, according to the A.L.A. (American Lung Association).

Keeping track with multiple inhalers and drugs may also be a pain, in addition to the cost of asthma medicines. You may be worried about finding an herbal remedy or holistic treatment for your asthma, whether you are searching for safe sources of asthma care or looking for ways to strengthen your asthma symptom management.

A variety of individuals with asthma are pursuing alternative therapy in order to enhance their asthma symptom regulation. Most individuals use alternative therapies, especially for allergic diseases.

About 40% of people with the condition of allergy are currently looking for a natural cure. "In accordance with conventional (treatment), often persons utilize it."

However, what does the study reveal regarding herbal treatments, and why do individuals owe them a shot? "Some of these have demonstrated advantages in animals as being anti-inflammatory,"

but in human trials, sadly, they have not really been proven to be successful.

While steam baths (warm) have also been used to aid relieve asthma-related nasal inflammation and airway pressure, it is pointed out that there has never been proof that steam therapies may ease asthma symptoms. It is important to remember that this is not an asthma treatment. Still, just because the study has not identified a definitive advantage doesn't mean that many individuals won't benefit from steam baths.

'Steam baths' can ease any of the effects as they provide the airways with moisture. Nevertheless, they warn that steam may be dangerously hot. However, they caution that steam may be dangerously hot. Steam baths can help to compensate for some symptoms, especially stuffiness of the nasal, but baths of steam are not "a replacement for medications of asthma."

Herbs & Other Asthma Alternative Treatment Options

A variety of herbs have been reported as natural asthma remedies, but it is recommended that when taking these asthma medications, individuals should be vigilant. These alternate therapeutic approaches and the related risks and incentives include:

Garlic

Thanks to its anti-inflammatory effects, garlic is used as a natural medication to treat many illnesses, especially heart disease. Since asthma disease is inflammatory, it might seem sensible that garlic might also be helpful in relieving the symptoms of asthma. However, it is reported that no laboratory studies have been undertaken exploring the impact of garlic on the symptoms of asthma. Hence, its function remains unclear in the management of asthma. However, the usage of garlic as an additional option for asthma is also being checked.

Ginger

It is also known to ease inflammation, and a new report has found that oral ginger extracts are associated with improving the symptoms of asthma.

However, the research did not indicate that ginger application contributed to any real change in lung function. It is therefore advised that this research be used as an alternative therapy for asthma to draw certain assumptions regarding the application of ginger. Further experiments are also being carried out in order to assess more closely whether ginger can regulate the effects of asthma more effectively.

Echinacea & the Licorice Root

One research investigating the usage of a variety of various herbs to combat asthma showed that not only was Echinacea, an herb frequently used to treat infections of the upper respiratory, unsuccessful, but it was also correlated with a variety of side effects. The complications involved with the usage of Echinacea are worsening asthma, skin rashes, and potential liver damage when combined with other drugs. Likewise, it has been found that licorice leaves, which have antioxidant and anti-inflammatory properties and are often used by people with asthma to soothe their lungs, are inadequate as a potential cure for asthma and are also correlated with adverse results such as high blood pressure. There are no clinical tests that both Echinacea and licorice root are effective treatments for asthma, and there have been several findings that in some people, Echinacea may worsen symptoms of asthma.

Stress

It can happen to anyone in these days to be stressed. Whether you are managing a full-time job, having a family, or just working on your own personal journey, the pressure of life can be overwhelming for some. It is not that stress is necessarily bad; it's the effects that stress has on you as an individual that you need to consider.

What is stress? It's the pressure that you feel in your life. And it is the response to this pressure that causes problems. Stress can multiply on top of itself, causing you to burn out and lose control. Stress has several negative effects on your body, leading to health problems down the line as well as making your psychological state a wreck.

But you can fight back. One of the biggest issues with stress is that it is very difficult for many people to recognize when they experience it nor do they know what to do about it.

Increased heart rate, elevated blood pressure, muscle tension, irritability, depression, stomachache, and indigestion are all signs of stress.

Turmeric

Turmeric has been the focus of a variety of experiments, and some anti-allergy properties have been identified. It is assumed that turmeric, which may induce inflammation, has an effect on histamines. However, before turmeric can be identified as a safe and efficient natural asthma treatment, more research must be performed.

Honey

Honey, used to help soothe an irritated throat & calm a cough, is an ingredient of many cold and cough remedies. There is no evidence to support its use as an alternative therapy for asthma symptoms, although many people with asthma may try to blend honey with a hot drink for relaxation.

Omega-3

Omega-3 fatty acids are also used as a natural therapy to avoid effectively and cure cardiovascular disease. Although some literature shows that omega-3s may also help minimize inflammation of the airway and improve lung capacity, there is still a great deal that is not understood regarding their role in the treatment of asthma.

To many people, stress means emotional stress. These (and other causes) make the body produce increased amounts of adrenaline.

This is how the body copes with stress. But the adrenaline release also causes the heart rate to increase, blood pressure to rise, and muscles to tense.

It's inevitable: you're going to face stress at some point in your life. Anybody who tells you they don't have it is either a liar or a robot. The important thing is to not let it get you down. Stress can be good for people—it can help them perform better on tests, in the workplace, and in social situations. Stress is inevitable, but it's also avoidable.

A host of conditions can develop when the body is subjected to prolonged stress. These include an increased rate of aging, reduced resistance to infection, weakened immune function (which, in turn, can lead to other conditions such as chronic fatigue syndrome), and hormone overproduction (which can lead to adrenal fatigue).

The best tool to fight off the effects of stress is a well-balanced diet and lifestyle.

Headache

Headache? Tired? Feeling a bit down? If you're feeling anything less than 100% today, you've probably heard of herbal remedies like peppermint to get your mind and body back on track. There's just one problem: many people don't know that there are also alternative treatments for physical ailments that come directly from Native American medicine.

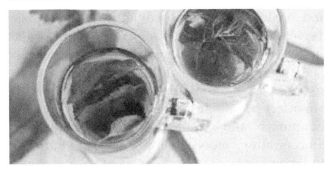

A headache is a pain in the head, sometimes just above the eyes. It can be caused by vigorous exercise, exposure to toxins, or it may result from symptoms that affect other parts of the body, such as eyestrain or diarrhea.

Different people feel different types of pain. Some feel a throbbing pain while others have a steady ache. Long-lasting headaches may involve fever and stiff neck muscles and are usually caused by sinus congestion.

Luckily, there are loads of easy-to-find herbs and other home remedies that can help with any problem. And the best part is because this knowledge has been passed down through generations (most often in a mother's language), it may be more suited to your specific needs than a Western approach.

Hangover

A hangover is a state that can manifest itself after heavy alcohol consumption. A hangover begins hours after the drinking concludes and is characterized by pain, fatigue, nausea, dizziness, and vomiting. Though there are many myths related to the best way to cure a hangover, there has been no scientific evidence proving any of them effective. The only known method of completely eliminating symptoms of a hangover is to drink enough water during and following drinking sessions until the individual beings urinating clear urine.

Hangovers are believed to be caused by the toxins acetaldehyde and methanol that are byproducts created when the body breaks down alcohol. Researchers believe these toxins cause inflammation of the cerebral cortex, nervous system, and stomach lining. As an alcoholic drink is absorbed into the body, a person's blood-alcohol content increases. Once this level becomes high enough, it slows down or stops vital functions, such as breathing and heart rate. After the alcohol has been consumed, it is absorbed into the bloodstream and distributed to all parts of the body through a process known as circulatory diffusion. Once the alcohol has diffused into the bloodstream, it is then broken down by an enzyme known as ADH (alcohol dehydrogenase). Although this enzyme breaks down alcohol effectively, it also creates two toxic byproducts- acetaldehyde and methanol. The brain has no means of removing these toxins from the bloodstream, which causes them to circulate throughout the body. In a process known as oxidation, these toxins create additional toxins that are eventually excreted in urine or sweat. Since some of these toxins remain in the body and inhibit vital functions related to brain function, it is commonly believed that the hangover is caused by poisoning.

Toxins aside, other factors contribute to a hangover. Alcohol can cause dehydration due to its diuretic effects. This may result in poor absorption of alcohol and slow the diffusion process, causing the feeling of a hangover. Other factors include heavy dieting, consumption of stimulants such as caffeine, and sleeping in an upright position (not lying on one's back). Although the most common factor is drinking large quantities of alcohol, this does not mean that excessive drinking causes a hangover. Some people who consume large quantities of alcohol during their lifetime may never experience a hangover because they have built up enough immunity to fight off those toxins.

Insomnia

Insomnia can be caused by a range of conditions but is most commonly seen as a difficulty in falling asleep, trouble staying asleep, or waking up too early in the morning. It has often been reported that individuals with insomnia experience disrupted patterns of sleep, delay going to bed at night, or have trouble dozing off when they want to be sleeping.

Signs and Symptoms

Insomnia symptoms include difficulty falling asleep at night and remaining asleep throughout the night; delayed onset of sleep; waking up too early in the morning; feeling wide awake/restless when you are trying to sleep; decreased quality and quantity of sleep over time.

Please note that the two main groups of insomnia are categorized as either subjective (having trouble falling asleep or waking up during the night) or objective (feeling rested but not refreshed upon waking up).

Sleep specialists usually diagnose primary insomnia when a person with no underlying medical condition has difficulty staying asleep or has difficulty falling asleep. It is also classified based on whether the symptoms last for at least one month. Insomnia itself is not a disease and can be caused by many factors, such as stress, depression, and anxiety. Medical conditions, such as major depressive disorder, sleep apnea, anxiety disorders, and post-traumatic stress disorder, are common causes of insomnia. Having trouble falling asleep is just one part of the spectrum of sleep problems that can affect people. Insomnia can cause many other symptoms and disorders, such as difficulty concentrating, mood changes, social withdrawal, and memory loss.

Insomnia is not a single disorder but rather a collection of many symptoms, all categorized under the umbrella term "insomnia." Insomnia is often divided into two separate sets according to whether the symptoms predominantly occur during the night (sleep) or daytime (wake).

Indigestion

Indigestion is caused by the accumulation of excessive amounts of stomach acid or hydrochloric acid in the stomach. The condition can also be caused by a bacterial infection, gastric ulcers, or an overgrowth of intestinal bacteria. Sometimes people experience chronic indigestion that results in the gradual destruction of their stomach tissues.

What Causes Indigestion?

Indigestion is typically caused by overeating; it can also be a side effect of certain medications such as aspirin and ibuprofen. These drugs lower the natural production of prostaglandins, which are hormones that protect the stomach lining from damage and regulate inflammation and blood flow. Excessive intake of aspirin and other NSAIDs can also cause gastrointestinal bleeding.

The duodenum is the main area of the small intestine where bacteria, chemicals, and digestive acids are produced before being absorbed into the

blood. Many people experience indigestion after consuming foods high in fat or protein or eating in a stressful situation such as travel; stress can affect the levels of hydrochloric acid produced by the stomach.

What Are the Symptoms?

Indigestion may lead to discomfort, bloating, and discomfort in one or more areas of the abdomen. A common symptom is a sensation that food is stuck somewhere in your throat. This may be accompanied by gas, burping, and sometimes vomiting. People with indigestion may also suffer from a general feeling of fatigue.

Menstrual Cycle Irregularities

The irregularities include various disruptions of the menstrual cycle. Each is addressed slightly differently, but a few overarching actions emerge that help with all of them: nourishing the body, improving circulation, and stimulating the liver and kidneys to clear away used-up hormones.

Delayed or absent menses may be due to a lack of adequate nourishment, especially protein, or disruptions in hormone levels. (Sometimes these share a cause. A high-sugar diet is nutrient-poor, and the havoc it wreaks on blood sugar levels has a cascade effect that disrupts hormone balance. Stress makes us tend to eat gratifying but poor-quality food and excessive stress-response hormones interfere with the normal actions of estrogen and progesterone). Irregular cycles, with no predictable pattern, may also be due to poor nourishment, liver stagnation or strain, or an irregular lifestyle, especially erratic sleep habits. The daily cycle shapes the monthly cycle, like small and large gears interlocking in a watch.

Over heavy bleeding generally comes from hormones not clearing efficiently at the liver, though it may also be connected with the development of fibroids or polyps. If heavy bleeding persists, seek medical attention.

Finally, let's talk about the most common menstrual ailment: dysmenorrhea, or menstrual pain, which usually begins just before menstruation, may occur in the lower abdomen or the lower back (and sometimes even into the thighs).

Other accompanying symptoms may include nausea, vomiting, headache, and either constipation or diarrhea.

There are two types of dysmenorrhea, primary and secondary. In primary dysmenorrhea, there is no underlying pain causing the disorder. It is thought that the pain occurs when uterine contractions reduce blood supply to the uterus. This may occur if the uterus is in the wrong position if the cervical opening is narrow, and a lack of exercise.

Secondary dysmenorrhea is when the pain is caused by some gynecological disorder, such as endometriosis (when the endometrium, the tissue that lines the uterus, abnormally grows on surfaces of other structures in the abdominal cavity), adenomyosis (in-growth of the endometrium into the uterine musculature), lesions, inflammation of the fallopian tubes, or uterine fibroids.

Also known as myomas, these masses occur in nearly one-quarter of all women by forty. Some women with uterine fibroids may have no symptoms. However, if symptoms are present, they include increased frequency of urination, a bloated feeling, pressure, pain, and abnormal bleeding.

Back Pain

Back pain is the most common type of pain experienced by people during their lifetime. Back pain occurs when some nerve or supporting structure in your back becomes irritated or inflamed. Depending on the cause, treatment can include medication, rest, physical therapy, and/or surgery.

Back Pain is one of the most widespread conditions affecting our society today. It causes a lot of discomfort for everyone and it also has a huge impact on many other personal aspects, such as work-life and quality of life. Several factors can cause back pain to start, including aging rather than having an accident that causes injury to your back muscles, ligaments, or joints.

Even though you may not be fully aware of the cause, back pain can happen at any time in your life.

It is important that you know some signs and symptoms to look for when you are experiencing back pain.

Signs of Back Pain

Pain when lifting or moving objects such as an item over your head or bending down to pick something up. Pain in your legs that feels like it comes from your hips or groin area when standing up straight. Pain that moves around in different areas and is triggered by different activities, such as sitting and standing in an only position. Sharp or cramping pains that occur after lying down (known as lying Down syndrome). Pain that is worse when you are cold or hungry and better when you eat or drink something. Pain that occurs in your buttocks, thighs, knees, and feet.

Bloating

Bloating, also known as abdominal distention, is the accumulation of gas within the stomach. A person who bloats might notice that their abdomen feels hardened and tight. The condition can be uncomfortable and painful.

The most common cause of bloating is drinking carbonated drinks such as soda or beer too quickly, eating lots of gas-producing foods like cabbage, beans, and broccoli (or other vegetables containing potassium), or being constipated for an extended period of time. Lots of water helps to relieve this problem. Some people who drink carbonated drinks too quickly, or eat foods that produce gas are unable to burp up the gas, and it gets trapped in the stomach.

As a result of the build-up of gas in the stomach, bloating can also be a symptom of other digestive disorders like irritable bowel syndrome (IBS), gastroesophageal reflux disease (GERD), and gastroparesis. Bloating has also been reported in patients with GERD after meals as an early symptom preceding other common GERD symptoms, such as heartburn, nausea, pain, or regurgitation.

Other causes of bloating could be ascites (fluid in the abdomen), a tumor, or infection in the abdomen. Several factors can cause hyperactive motility in the stomach muscle.

In many cases, bloating can be relieved with medication or medical treatment. Although there is no single cause or course for bloat, many people appear to find relief within days to weeks by taking an over-the-counter laxative, dieting, avoiding gas-producing foods, and drinking less carbonated soda. Other gastrointestinal conditions may require medical treatment, including surgery if no medical treatment is successful.

The Relevant Tissue States

- Dampness (stagnation).

Relevant Herbal Actions

- Carminative.
- Lymphatic.

Herbal Allies

- Angelica.
- Calendula flower.
- Fennel seed.
- Ginger.
- Peppermint leaf.
- Self-heal leaf and flower.

Bloating may be extremely common, but it's not insignificant! When you become bloated, it's a buildup of gas in the bowels or a flood of fluid swelling in the lymphatic vessels wrapped around the intestines. Fennel and ginger are great for reducing gas, but for fluid bloating, you'll want lymphatic drainers such as calendula or self-heal.

Bronchitis/Chest Cold/Pneumonia

There are three types of respiratory illnesses that cause coughing and chest pain: bronchitis, pneumonia, and the common cold. Bronchitis is an infection of the lungs that starts in the airways. Pneumonia is a lung infection that can come from a virus or bacteria. A common cold virus may lead to a sinus infection or ear infection, which can cause coughing and pain in your chest. Coughs in babies and children are often caused by a cold.

Coughing can become a problem for children for several reasons. Hyperactive children, who have difficulty settling down and concentrating, may cough due to increased mucus production caused by infection, allergy, or postnasal drip. Nursing mothers who smoke or are exposed to secondhand smoke experience a higher incidence of childhood asthma, ear infections, and bronchitis. Pacifier use is also associated with more respiratory infections in babies.

The Relevant Tissue States

- Dampness.
- Cold (depressed vitality).

Relevant Herbal Actions

- Antimicrobial.
- Astringent.

- Decongestant.
- Diaphoretic.
- Expectorant.
- Pulmonary tonic.

Herbal Allies

- Angelica.
- Elder.
- Elecampane root.
- Garlic.
- Ginger.
- Pine.
- Sage leaf.
- Thyme leaf.

When you have a lung infection, don't suppress the cough, it's a vital response! Our goal is to cough when it's productive, so all the irritating or infectious material is expelled as you cough up phlegm, and to reduce the amount of unproductive coughing. If you can't bring up the phlegm, you may find a simple cough developing into pneumonia because of the mucus buildup. (True pneumonia is serious conditions seek higher care. Meanwhile, take elecampane and garlic they're your strongest allies for this problem). Infection-instigated coughs are usually wet, and the herbs we discuss here assume that's the case. Refer to cough for more help to determine what kind of cough you have. The goal is to get it just a little on the moist side—nice and productive—so you can expel that phlegm.

As with any respiratory condition, herbal steam is a great remedy all on its own, combating infection and greatly improving blood circulation—which means immune activity—in the lungs. Simple steam with thyme or sage is very good for this problem.

Burns and Sunburn

Aburn occurs when our skin is exposed to heat or radiation (including infrared radiation) and may be considered superficial if the heat reaches only the outer layers of skin (epidermis). However, if our deeper layers of skin are damaged (the dermal layer), then it's classified as first or second-degree burns. If we're particularly unlucky and both epidermis and dermal layers are hurt, then it could be considered third-degree burns.

Sunburns are a type of superficial burn, caused by prolonged exposure to UV radiation. These occur in the exposed areas of skin, especially the face, neck, and arms.

The Relevant Tissue States

- Heat.

Relevant Herbal Actions

- Anti-inflammatory.
- Antimicrobial.
- Antiseptic.
- Vulnerary.

Herbal Allies

- Calendula flower.
- Linden leaf and flower.
- Marshmallow.
- Peppermint leaf.
- Plantain leaf.
- Rose petals.
- Self-heal leaf and flower.

Immediately following a burn, run cold water over the area—the skin retains heat for much longer than you'd expect. (If blisters form in the burned area, be very gentle with them and don't break them before they naturally slough off, if you can avoid it.) Then, gently clean the wound, removing any dirt or contaminant. Apply the herbs, combining antiseptics to prevent infection with cooling, wound-healing herbs to encourage tissue regeneration.

Apply any of the herbal allies in a wash, compress, poultice, or infused honey—don't use oily preparations (like slaves) on burns because they trap the heat in the tissue.

Do not underestimate the power of a marshmallow root poultice! Simply saturate a handful of marshmallow roots with enough cold water to make a sticky mass and apply it to the burn. Cover with gauze and leave in place for 20 minutes. Repeat frequently.

Cholesterol Management

Cholesterol is a type of fat found in your blood and in some of your organs. Cholesterol helps to keep the inner walls of your cells healthy, but too much cholesterol can lead to health problems like heart disease.

Guidelines on how much cholesterol you need each day vary depending on factors like which country you live in and whether you are an adult older than age 50. The American Heart Association suggests a limit of 300 milligrams (<200 mg/day for people with certain health conditions) per day, while the National Institutes of Health suggest eating less than 300 mg (<200 mg/day for people with certain health conditions) per day to avoid developing heart disease.

Your body does not make cholesterol, which means you must get it from your diet. Good sources of cholesterol include animal products like egg yolks, organ meats, poultry skin, and whole milk. The amount of cholesterol in animal products varies depending on the cuts of meat or if the meat comes from a farm-raised fish. For example, steak has more than twice as much cholesterol as chicken breast fillets.

Vegetable oils and fats are also rich in cholesterol. These include things like lard, palm oil, and coconut oil. 2 tablespoons of butter or margarine provide about 100 milligrams of cholesterol, while one tablespoon of vegetable shortening provides about 30 milligrams. You should get about 10%–15% of your daily calories from fat, so try to limit your cholesterol intake to that level.

The Relevant Tissue States

- Heat (inflammation).

Teeth and Mouth Ailments

One of the most common but also one of the most unpleasant dental concerns is tooth decay. This is caused by acids produced by bacteria in your mouth when certain sugars and starches dissolve into your saliva. The process can be greatly sped up if you eat food with high sugar content or drink

Relevant Herbal Actions

- Anti-inflammatory.
- Antioxidant.
- Hepatic.
- Hypotensive.

Herbal Allies

- Cinnamon bark.
- Garlic.
- Ginger.
- Kelp.
- Linden leaf and flower.
- Rose.
- Yarrow leaf and flower.

High cholesterol is a symptom, not a freestanding problem. It is an indicator that systemic inflammation is damaging the blood vessels. Many things can cause this blood sugar dysregulation. Insufficient sleep and stress are major factors, but the biggest one is diet.

Herbal approaches to reducing cholesterol levels primarily rely on the antioxidant power of the plants to reduce inflammation and neutralize free radicals.

Garlic is one of the most well-known and extensively studied herbs for reducing inflammation in the blood vessels. Adding it to your food is a simple and effective way to lower cholesterol levels and improve other blood parameters beneficial effects start to manifest with amounts as low as two garlic cloves per day.

sweetened beverages such as juice or soda, which can cause a lot of damage to tooth enamel over time.

Additionally, gum disease that progresses to periodontitis—inflammation, and infection of gums—happens particularly when there are not enough teeth left with healthy enamel to support strong gum tissue. This kind of condition increases the risk of bone loss and, in severe cases, tooth loss. The problem is that many people are not even aware of gum disease until they begin to experience pain while chewing or notice that their gums bleed very easily.

Out of Sight, Out of Mind

It turns out that we are quite efficient at ignoring oral health problems, which might not seem like a big deal until you consider how many functions your mouth and teeth play in your life. Aside from eating and talking, your mouth houses the mechanism for making facial expressions and smells. If you lose the function of any one tooth, you may not realize its significance until a different part of your body begins to hurt because your jaw cannot chew properly or other teeth have collapsed due to poor alignment.

Gingivitis is an inflammation of the gum tissue. It manifests as reddening, swelling, and at times, bleeding of the gums. The cause of gingivitis is the accumulation of plaque on teeth, and its removal will almost certainly reverse the disease. If untreated, gingivitis can lead to gingival shrinkage and loose teeth.

An abscess is a different kettle of fish. It is a more severe condition related to a serious bacterial infection, which causes the production of pus.

Abscesses can appear anywhere in the body: folliculitis, whitlows, and mouth abscesses are the most common forms. They manifest as swelling,

- Uva ursi leaves.
- Yarrow leaves.
- Plantain leaves.
- Heal all leaves and flowers.
- Calendula flowers.
- Licorice root.
- Barberry fruit and leaves.
- White oak bark and leaves.
- Echinacea root.
- Oregon grape root.
- Lizard tail root.
- Sage leaves.
- Thyme leaves.
- Goldenrod leaves and flowers.

heat, and a reddening of the part (like pimples) and are often accompanied by fever.

Antibiotics are the common medical treatment for them but, as you will probably know, they are like an insecticide: they destroy everything in their path, from the germs that cause the infection to the intestinal bacterial flora (that is essential to our digestion), the white blood cells (who fight the infections), and the lymphocytes (who produce the antibodies).

Herbs could help you effectively fight infections and inflammation without these side effects from this point of view.

Finally, Canker Sores are small sores that can appear on lips, tongue, and throat. They present as white or yellow ulcers surrounded by inflamed tissue.

The causes of canker sores may be a viral infection, poor dental hygiene, or lack of vitamins and nutrients.

Symptomatology

- Inflammation and laxity of the tissue.

Actions Required

- Anti-inflammatory.
- Antibacterial.
- Astringent.

Recommended Herbs

- Chamomile.

Part IX

~

Herbal Recipes

Aging Remedies

Anti-Aging Tea

Preparation time: 5 minutes.

Cooking time: 3 minutes.

Servings: 1

Ingredients:

- 1 teaspoon dandelion root
- 1 teaspoon burdock root
- 1 teaspoon schisandra berries
- 1 tablespoon nettle leaves
- 1 teaspoon hibiscus flowers, dried
- 1 teaspoon chamomile-extract
- 1/2 cup of water

Directions:

1. Fill a pan halfway with water and bring to a boil.
2. Combine all the ingredients and steep for two to three minutes.
3. Transfer to a cup and enjoy.

Lung-strengthening Remedies

If you're struggling with asthma, you'll be happy to know that there are some natural ways of relieving your symptoms. Here are some easy home remedies which may help.

- **Lung-strengthening tea:** make tea by boiling 2 leaves of licorice root in a pot for 10 minutes. Steep it in boiling water for about 15 minutes and drink without sweeteners or milk (unless you're following Ayurvedic medicine).

- **Lung-strengthening tincture:** take 1 tablespoon of dried licorice root and pour over 1 cup of apple cider vinegar (make sure the cup is at least 8 ounces). Let it steep for at least a week, then strain the liquid and pour into a dropper bottle. Take 1 drop in water 3 times daily.

- **Lung-strengthening pills:** boil the aforementioned herbs (1/2 teaspoon of each) in 1 cup of water for about 5 minutes. Turn off heat and let steep for at least an hour. Pour into a blender with 1/2 cup of yogurt and blend well. This can be used to make lung-strengthening pills, which are taken as needed.

- **Lung-strengthening ointment:** combine equal parts of canola oil and petroleum jelly. Apply it at bedtime for asthma and allergies.

Stress remedies

Calm Down Tea

Preparation time: 10 minutes.

Cooking time: 30 minutes.

Servings: 2

Ingredients:

- 1 teaspoon powdered ginger
- 1 teaspoon powdered valerian root
- 1 teaspoon powdered pleurisy root
- 2 cups boiling water

Directions:

1. Combine the above herbs in a nonmetallic container and cover with boiling water; steep for 30 minutes; cool and strain.

2. Take one tablespoon at a time, as needed, up to two cups a day.

Shake-It-Off Tea

Preparation time: 10 minutes.

Cooking time: 30 minutes.

Servings: 2

Ingredients:

- 1 to 2 teaspoons peppermint leaves
- 1 teaspoon valerian root
- 1 cup boiling water

Directions:

1. Combine the above ingredients and cover with boiling water; steep for 20 to 30 minutes; strain.

2. Drink up to one cup per day, as needed.

Cooling Headache Tea

Preparation time: 10 minutes.

Cooking time: 10 minutes.

Servings: 2

Ingredients:

- 2 tablespoons fresh mint leaves, roughly chopped
- 1 tablespoon fresh thyme leaves, finely chopped
- 1 teaspoon anise seeds, crushed in a mortar or zested from a lemon in a spice grinder

- 5 cups boiling water or 1.5L cold water plus ice cubes.

Directions:

1. Bring 5 cups of boiling water or 1.5 liters of cold tea to a full rolling boil and pour over the herbs and let steep for 2 minutes before straining into your desired mug or cup. Add ice cubes to make it more refreshing if desired. Drink while still hot or enjoy at any temperature by adding ice.

The medicinal properties of mint are known to help with headaches.

According to some research, the menthol and other volatile oils in mint may act as natural painkillers by inhibiting the release of pro-inflammatory neuropeptides from sensory nerves, and by blocking pain signals to the brain

Headache Remedies

Warming Headache Tea

Preparation time: 5 minutes.

Cooking time: 10 minutes.

Servings: 2

Ingredients

- 1 tablespoon Cinnamon
- 2 Cloves
- 1 tablespoon Ginger
- 1 tablespoon Cayenne pepper flakes
- 2 Tea bags
- Water (about 2 cups)

Directions:

1. Add about 4 tablespoons of water to a small pot and bring it to a boil.
2. Add the tea bags, spices, and cayenne pepper flakes and allow boiling for about 5 minutes straight. Remove from heat just before the tea turns black or becomes bitter.

Allow the tea to cool slightly before drinking it cold or adding honey for sweetness as desired. Drink once a day until symptoms disappear or on an as-needed basis if pain persists after other treatments have been attempted with no success in relieving symptoms.

Peppery Headache Tea

Preparation time: 5 minutes.

Cooking time: 10 minutes.

Servings: 2

Ingredients:

- 1 tablespoon ginger
- 1 teaspoon dried pepper pods
- 1-liter water

Directions:

Bring water to a boil, turn the heat off, and add everything. Cover and steep for 5 minutes. Strain, enjoy!

Hangover Remedies

Hangover Tea 1

Preparation time: 15 minutes.

Cooking time: 5 minutes.

Servings: 1

Ingredients:

- 1 teaspoon catnip dried leaves
- 1 teaspoon peppermint dried leaves
- 1 teaspoon barberry dried leaves
- 1 cup distilled boiling water

Directions:

Pour boiling water over the herbs mixture. Let rest for 30 minutes. Strain and drink.

Hangover Tea 2

Preparation time: 5 minutes.

Cooking time: 5 minutes.

Servings: 1

Ingredients:

- 1 teaspoon barberry dried leaves
- 1 teaspoon heal-all dried leaves
- 1 teaspoon Oregon grape root
- 1 cup distilled boiling water

Directions:

Pour boiling water over the herbs mixture. Let rest for half an hour. Strain and drink throughout the day.

Hangover Tea 3

Preparation time: 10 minutes.

Cooking time: 6 minutes.

Servings: 1

Ingredients:

- 1 teaspoon barberry dried leaves
- 1 teaspoon goldenseal dried leaves
- 1 teaspoon Oregon grape root
- 1 cup distilled boiling water

Directions:

Pour boiling water over the herbs mixture. Let rest for half an hour. Strain and drink throughout the day.

Hangover Tea 4

Preparation time: 12 minutes.

Cooking time: 6 minutes.

Servings: 1

Ingredients:

- 1 tablespoon plantain dried leaf
- 1 tablespoon calendula dried flower
- 1 tablespoon chamomile dried flower
- 1 tablespoon dried linden leaves
- 1 tablespoon licorice root
- 1 tablespoon dried ginger root
- 1 tablespoon dried St. john's wort leaves

Directions:

Mix the herbs in a mason jar for easy storage. Put 1 tablespoon of the mixture in 1 cup of distilled boiling water. Let rest for half an hour. Strain and drink throughout the day.

Fast-Acting Hangover Tea

Preparation time: 9 minutes.

Cooking time: 5 minutes.

Servings: 1

Ingredients:

- 1 green tea bag
- 1 cup of water

Directions:

1. In a saucepan, add the water and let it warm.
2. Then add all the green tea bags to a mug and pour the boiled water over it.
3. Lest it steep for five minutes, then enjoy!

Insomnia Remedies

End-of-the-Day Elixir

Preparation time: 10 minutes.

Cooking time: 10 minutes

Servings: 4 fluid ounces (60 to 120 doses).

This blend of relaxants and gentle sedatives doesn't force sleep but helps relieve the tension, anxiety, and distraction that make it difficult to transition into sleep. This formula (and any herbs taken to aid in sleep) is best taken in "Pulse doses," which is much more effective than taking the total dose all at once right at bedtime. It gives the herbs time to start working in your system and emphasizes to the body that it's time to transition into sleep.

Ingredients:

- 1 fluid ounce tincture of chamomile 1 fluid ounce tincture of betony
- ¾ fluid ounce tincture of ashwagandha
- ½ fluid ounce tincture of catnip
- ½ fluid ounce tincture of linden
- ¼ fluid ounce honey (plain or rose petal–infused)

Directions:

1. In a small bottle, combine the tinctures and honey. Cap the bottle and label it.
2. One hour before bedtime, take 1 to 2 drops.
3. Thirty minutes before bedtime, take another 1 to 2 drops.
4. At bedtime, take the final 1 to 2 drops.

Sleep! Formula

Preparation time: 10 minutes.

Cooking time: 20 minutes

Servings: 4 fluid ounces (60 to 120 doses).

For this formula, we recruit wild lettuce, the strongest hypnotic (sleep-inducing) herb, in this chapter. This is especially helpful if part of what's keeping you up at night is physical pain, as wild lettuce also has a pain-relieving effect. This formula, like End-of-the-Day Elixir, is best taken in "pulse doses."

Ingredients:

- 2 fluid ounces tincture of wild lettuce
- 1 fluid ounce tincture of betony

- ½ fluid ounce tincture of chamomile
- ½ fluid ounce tincture of linden

Directions:

1. In a small bottle, combine the tinctures. Cap the bottle and label it.
2. One hour before bedtime, take 1 to 2 drops.
3. Thirty minutes before bedtime, take another 1 to 2 drops. At bedtime, take the final 1 to 2 drops.

Insomnia Relief Tea

Preparation time: 10 minutes.

Cooking time: 30 minutes.

Servings: 2

Ingredients:

- 1 teaspoon chamomile flowers
- 1 teaspoon hops
- 1 teaspoon valerian root
- 1 cup boiling water

Directions:

1. Combine the above herbs.
2. Take one tablespoon of the mixture and cover with boiling water; let steep for 30 minutes; strain.
3. Drink warm, as needed, half a cup at a time.

Sweet Dreams Tea

Preparation time: 5 minutes

Cooking time: 30 minutes

Servings: 2

Ingredients:

- 2 teaspoons catnip leaves
- 1 teaspoon hops
- 2 teaspoons chamomile flower
- 2 teaspoons passionflower
- 1 cup boiling water

Directions:

1. Combine the above herbs in a glass container; cover with boiling water; steep for 30 minutes; cool and strain.

Indigestion Remedies
Digestive Tea 1
Preparation time: 10 minutes.

Cooking time: 20 minutes.

Servings: 1

Ingredients:

- 1 teaspoon licorice root dried, powder
- 1 Teaspoon peppermint dried leaves
- 1 cup distilled boiling water

Directions:

1. Pour boiling water over the herbs. Let steep for 20 minutes. Strain and drink warm to help digestion.

Digestive Tea 2
Preparation time: 10 minutes

Cooking time: 30 minutes

Servings: 1

Ingredients:

- 1 teaspoon ginger root dried
- 1 teaspoon angelica root dried
- 1 teaspoon chamomile dried flowers
- 1 teaspoon peppermint dried leaves
- 1 cup distilled boiling water

Directions:

1. Pour boiling water over the herbs mixture. Let rest for half an hour. Strain and drink.

Digestive Tea 3
Preparation time: 5 minutes.

Cooking time: 30 minutes.

Servings: 1

Ingredients:

- 1 teaspoon black cohosh root dried
- 1 teaspoon angelica root dried

2. Take one hour before bedtime.

- 1 cup distilled boiling water

Directions:

1. Pour boiling water over the herbs mixture. Let rest for 30 minutes. Strain and drink throughout the day to help with persistent indigestion.

Intestinal Gas Tincture
Preparation time: 15 minutes.

Cooking time: 0 minutes.

Servings: 1

Ingredients:

- 3 tablespoons fennel seed tincture
- 3 tablespoons ginger root tincture
- 3 tablespoons licorice root tincture
- 3 tablespoons peppermint tincture
- 3 tablespoons chamomile flowers tincture

Directions:

1. Put the tinctures in an amber glass bottle with a dropper lid in the indicated proportions. Label it. Take 5 drops after each meal.

Preventive Tincture
Preparation time: 15 minutes.

Cooking time: 0 minutes.

Servings: 1

Ingredients:

- 3 tablespoons fennel seed tincture
- 3 tablespoons dandelion root tincture
- 3 tablespoons licorice root tincture
- 3 tablespoons sage leaves tincture

Directions:

1. Put the tinctures in an amber glass bottle with a dropper lid in the indicated

proportions. Label it. Take 3 drops before each meal.

Menstrual Cycle Irregularities Remedies

Steady Cycle Tea

Preparation time: 20 minutes.

Cooking time: 0 minutes.

Servings: 2

These herbs provide substantial nourishment and a bit of gentle kidney, lymphatic, and endocrine stimulation. Long-term use of a formula like this has been the major factor in improving many of our clients with menstrual irregularities of all types. Add ginger if you run cold, betony if you're frequently anxious, and peppermint for taste (if you like it). Drink a quart or more every day.

Ingredients:

- 1 cup dried nettle leaf
- 1 cup dried dandelion leaf
- ½ cup dried goldenrod leaf and flower
- ½ cup dried self-heal leaf and flower
- ¼ cup dried tulsi leaf
- ¼ cup dried kelp

Directions:

1. In a small bowl, mix all the herbs. Store in an airtight container.

2. Make a long infusion: Prepare a kettle of boiling water. Measure 2 to 3 tablespoons of herbs per quart of water and place in a Mason jar or French press. Pour in the boiling water, cover, and steep for 8 hours or overnight.

3. Makes 3(½) cups dried herb mix (enough for 20 to 28 quarts of tea).

Bleed On! Tea

Preparation time: 20 minutes.

Cooking time: 20 minutes.

Servings: 3 cups dried herb mix (enough for 20 to 26 quarts of tea).

To bring on menstruation, drink this tea for 3 days to 1 week before the expected start of your next period. Drink this tea very hot for the best results. Reheat as necessary and drink a quart or more over the day. For a stronger effect, take a drop of angelica tincture together with each cup of tea.

Ingredients:

- 1 cup dried chamomile flower
- 1 cup dried tulsi leaf
- ⅓ cup dried goldenrod leaf and flower
- ⅓ cup dried ginger
- ⅓ cup dried angelica root

Directions:

1. In a small bowl, mix all the herbs. Store in an airtight container.

2. Make a hot infusion: Prepare a kettle of boiling water. Measure 2 to 3 tablespoons of herbs per quart of water and place in a Mason jar or French press. Pour in the boiling water, cover, and steep for 20 minutes or until cool enough to drink.

Daily Soothing Menstrual Tea

Preparation time: 10 minutes.

Cooking time: 0 minutes.

Servings: 4

Ingredients:

- 2 teaspoons black haw root or bark
- 2 teaspoons passionflower
- 2 cups cold water

Directions:

1. Combine the above herbs in a pan and cover with cold water; soak overnight; strain.

2. Take half a cup, up to four times daily.

Back Pain Remedies

Spine's Fine Tincture

Preparation time: 10 minutes.

Cooking time: 0 minutes.

Servings: 2

Servings: 4 fluid ounces (40 to 120 doses).

These warming, relaxant, analgesic herbs quell the spasms responsible for most back pain, regardless of whether the pain is acute or chronic, muscular or connective, etc. If you have infused oil made from fresh goldenrod or ginger, use it as massage oil after applying this formula topically. To help sleep, take 1 to 4 drops of tincture of wild lettuce orally, this will also contribute more pain-relieving action.

Ingredients

- 1 fluid ounce tincture of Solomon's seal
- 1 fluid ounce tincture of ginger
- ½ fluid ounce tincture of goldenrod
- ½ fluid ounce tincture of meadowsweet
- ½ fluid ounce tincture of mullein root (see Tip)
- ½ fluid ounce tincture of St. John's wort (optional; see Tip)

Directions

1. Take 1 to 4 drops by mouth 3 to 5 times per day.
2. Additionally, pour 1 to 4 drops into your palm and rub them into the back muscles.
3. **Tip:** If the vertebral discs are impinged or worn away, increase the mullein root to 1 fluid ounce. It specifically supports these tissues. If sciatica or other radiating nerve pain is present, include St. John's wort

Bloating Remedies

Dispersing Infusion

Preparation time: 10 minutes.

Cooking time: 20 minutes.

Servings: 3 to 3½ cups dried herb mix (enough for 18 to 24 quarts of tea).

This helps with bloating, no matter what kind. Feel free to adjust the proportions to your taste, and if you don't have every herb, it is still effective. **Be**

(unless you are taking pharmaceuticals). It regenerates damaged nerve tissue.

Nutrition:

- **Protein:** 12% 29 kcal
- **Fat:** 16% 25 kcal
- **Carbohydrates:** 72% 122 kcal

Ming Compress

Makes 1 compress. This simple application provides immediate relief.

Ingredients

- 16 fluid ounces water
- ½ cup dried ginger (see tip)
- ¼ cup Epsom salts

Directions

1. In a small pot with a tight-fitting lid over high heat, combine all the ingredients. Cover and bring to a boil. Reduce the heat and simmer for 5 minutes. Meanwhile, fill a hot water bottle.
2. Soak a cloth in the hot tea, holding it in a dry spot and letting it cool in the air until hot but comfortable to the touch.
3. Lie down and place the wet cloth over your back. Cover with a dry cloth and lay the hot water bottle on top. Get comfortable and let it soak in for 10 to 20 minutes. You should feel warmth, relaxation, and relief from pain.
4. Repeat as often as desired.

Tip: Have pain, but no dried ginger? If all you have on hand is fresh ginger from the grocery store, you can use that, too sliced, chopped, or grated.

forewarned: This will induce you to pass on some gas!

Ingredients:

- 1 cup dried calendula flower
- 1 cup dried self-heal leaf and flower
- ½ cup fennel seed
- ½ cup dried ginger
- ½ cup dried peppermint leaf (optional)

Directions:

1. In a medium bowl, mix together all the herbs, including the peppermint (if using). Store in an airtight container.

2. Make hot implantation: Prepare a pot of bubbling water. Measure 2 to 3 tablespoons of spices for each quart of water and spot in a Mason container or French press. Pour in the bubbling water, cover, and steep for 20 minutes or until sufficiently cool to drink.

3. Drink 1 to 2 teacups after meals to prevent or dispel bloating. If this is a chronic issue, drink a quart or more every day.

Dispersing Tincture
Preparation time: 10 minutes.

Cooking time: 0 minutes.

Bronchitis Remedies
Fire Cider
Preparation time: 30 minutes.

Cooking time: 0 minutes.

Servings: about 1-quart.

Traditional fire cider recipes are blends of spicy and aromatic stimulating expectorants that will heat you and help you get the gunk out. In this version, we sneak in some immune stimulants and a good source of vitamin C. Do not consume this if you take pharmaceutical blood thinners.

Ingredients:

- 1 whole head garlic, cloves peeled and chopped
- 1 (2-inch) piece fresh ginger, chopped
- ¼ cups dried pine needles
- ¼ cup dried sage leaf
- ¼ cup dried thyme leaf
- ¼ cup dried elderberry
- ¼ cups dried raised hips
- 2 tablespoons dried elecampane root

Servings: 4 fluid ounces (60 to 120 doses).

A few drops of this tincture mixture will disperse gas and fluid bloating alike. Bring it with you the next time you head out for pizza or go to the local diner, and pass it around after the meal!

Ingredients:

- 1 fluid ounce tincture of calendula
- 1 fluid ounce tincture of self-heal
- 1 fluid ounce tincture of fennel
- ½ fluid ounce tincture of ginger
- ½ fluid ounce tincture of angelica

Directions:

1. 1. In a small bottle, combine the tinctures. Cap the bottle and label it.

2. Take 1 to 2 drops as needed.

- 2 tablespoons dried angelica root
- 1-quart apple cider vinegar
- Honey or water, for sweetening or diluting (optional)

Directions:

1. Fill the jar with vinegar. Cover the jar with a plastic lid, or place a sheet of wax paper under the jar lid before you screw down the ring. (The coating on the bottom of metal Mason jar lids corrodes when exposed to vinegar).

2. Let the herbs macerate in the vinegar for 2 weeks or longer.

3. Strain, bottle, and label the finished fire cider. If the vinegar is too heating to be comfortable on your stomach, add some honey (up to one-fourth the total volume), or dilute your dose with water.

Take a shot (about ½ fluid ounce) at the first sign of mucus buildup in the lungs, and every couple of hours thereafter until symptoms resolve.

Sunburn Remedies

Burn-Healing Honey

Preparation time: 10 minutes.

Cooking time: 0 minutes.

Servings: about 1-pint.

Honey is the single best healing agent for burns: If you have nothing but plain honey, you're still in good shape. It gets even better, though, when you infuse these healing herbs into it ahead of time.

Ingredients:

- ½ cup fresh calendula flower
- ½ cup fresh rose petals
- 1-pint honey, gently warmed

Sunburn Spray

Preparation time: 20 minutes.

Cooking time: 20 minutes.

Servings: 8 fluid ounces.

A few spritzes cool the skin and begin to reduce inflammation.

Ingredients:

- 1 tablespoon dried peppermint leaf
- 1 tablespoon dried plantain leaf
- 1 tablespoon dried self-heal leaf and flower
- 1 tablespoon dried linden leaf and flower
- 1-quart boiling water
- 4 fluid ounces of rose water

Directions:

Cholesterol Remedies

Antioxidant Tea

Preparation time: 10 minutes.

Cooking time: 20 minutes.

Servings: about 2 cups dried herb mix (enough for 12 to 16 quarts of tea).

Gentle linden helps soften and direct the other herbs in this blend, focusing their effects on the blood vessels to improve integrity and reduce inflammation. Drink a quart or more of this tea every day.

Ingredients:

Directions:

1. Put the calendula and raised petals in a pint-size mason jar.

2. Fill the jar with warm honey. Seal the jar and place it in a warm area to infuse for 1 month.

3. In a double boiler, gently warm the closed jar until the honey has a liquid consistency. Strain the infused honey into a new jar, pressing against the strainer to extract as much honey as you can.

4. After cooling and cleaning a burn site, apply a layer of the infused honey and cover lightly with a gauze bandage. Refresh the application at least twice a day.

1. Make a hot infusion: In a mason jar, combine the peppermint, plantain, self-heal, and linden. Pour in the boiling water, cover, and steep for 20 minutes.

2. Move the jar to the refrigerator until it's cold.

3. Strain out 4 fluid ounces of the infusion and transfer to an 8-ounce bottle with a fine-mist sprayer top. Use the remaining infusion for compresses or a cooling drink. It will keep refrigerated for 3 days.

4. Add the rose water to the spray bottle. Cap the bottle and label it.

5. Apply copiously and frequently. Keep the spray refrigerated when not in use.

- 1 cup dried linden leaf and flower
- ½ cup dried raised petals, hips, or a combination
- ¼ cup dried cinnamon bark
- ¼ cup dried yarrow leaf and flower
- 1 tablespoon dried ginger

Directions:

1. In a medium bowl, mix all the herbs. Store in an airtight container.

2. Make a hot mixture: Prepare a pot of bubbling water. Measure 2 to 3 tablespoons of spices for each quart of water and spot in a Mason container or French press. Pour in the bubbling water, cover, and steep for 20 minutes or until sufficiently cool to drink.

Rose Hip Quick Jam

Preparation time: 20 minutes.

Cooking time: 1 hour.

Servings: about 3 ounces (2 servings).

This simple, tasty treat is a powerhouse of vitamin C, bioflavonoids, and antioxidant goodness. Mix this into your oatmeal or other hot cereal, spread it on toast, or just eat it with a spoonful!

Ingredients

- 2 tablespoons dried rosehips
- 2 fluid ounces water
- 1 teaspoon honey
- 1 teaspoon powdered cinnamon

Directions

1. In a cup or small bowl, stir together the rosehips and water. Let sit for about 1 hour, so the rosehips soften and absorb the water.

1. They'll get into a jam-like substance.

2. Stir in the honey and cinnamon.

Prepare fresh each day for maximum potency.

Teeth and Mouth Aliments Remedies

Anti-Inflammatory Mouthwash

Preparation time: 10 minutes.

Cooking time: 0 minutes.

Servings : 2

Ingredients:

- 8 ounces distilled water
- 2 teaspoons Epsom salt
- 2 ounces Uva ursi tincture
- 2 ounces yarrow tincture
- 1-ounce plantain tincture
- 1-ounce heal-all tincture
- 1-ounce calendula tincture
- ½ ounces heal-all tincture
- ½ ounces licorice tincture

Directions:

1. Combine all the ingredients above in a glass container.

2. After brushing your teeth, take a mouthful of the mouthwash and swish for about 4 minutes.

Anti-Abscess Mouthwash

Preparation time: 10 minutes.

Cooking time: 30 minutes.

Servings : 1

Ingredients:

- 20 ounces distilled boiling water
- 4 tablespoons barberries
- 4 tablespoons oak bark
- 4 teaspoons Echinacea root
- 4 teaspoons Oregon grape root powdered

Directions:

1. Combine all the ingredients above in a glass container. Let it rest for 6 hours before straining.

2. After brushing your teeth, take a mouthful of the mouthwash and swish for about 4 minutes.

Anti-Abscess Tea

Preparation time: 10 minutes.

Cooking time: 0 minutes.

Servings : 5

Ingredients:

- ¼ ounces Echinacea tincture
- ½ ounces lizard tail root tincture
- 25 ounces distilled water

Directions:

Heat the water and put the tinctures in it. Makes 5 cups to drink throughout the day.

Part X

~

Herbal Remedies for Children

Bites and Stings

There are many types of stings or bites you may get from allergies, bee or wasp stings, mosquitoes, biting flies, ticks, caterpillars, and spiders. Bites from these insects can cause an infection. Most people don't have much experience with insect bites and stings as they are often associated with little kids who play outside too much.

These are not usually serious infections; however, some can cause a great deal of itching and swelling. If you have had more than one bite or sting in a short space of time, then you should always see your doctor and get medical attention.

Bites from insects are generally very similar to bites from other animals. The main difference is that insect venom doesn't contain proteins in the same way as other venomous creatures, such as snakes or spiders, so it rarely causes the more severe allergic reactions that snake and spider venom can cause. However, an allergic reaction to any insect bite or sting, such as hives or swelling, could prove extremely serious and life-threatening if associated with other allergic symptoms such as asthma or anaphylaxis.

If the area is very itchy and sore, this could be because the venom has already entered the bloodstream and there are bigger problems to deal with. If possible, don't scratch any itchy areas as this can spread the venom further into your system.

If you have been stung or bitten by an insect, keep an eye on the area. If it gets worse instead of better in the next few hours, or if the symptoms are affecting different parts of your body, then you should always seek medical attention. As well as redness and swelling, symptoms to look out for can include:

- Swelling around the mouth and/or facial area.
- Difficulty swallowing.
- Difficulty breathing.
- Swelling of other parts of the body, such as hands, feet, and ankles. If a swollen limb becomes pale or tinged with blue, then this means that there is not enough blood flowing through the area and it could be due to shock causing a loss of circulation.
- Pain or redness at the site of the bite.
- Numbness and/or tingling around the bite.
- Any persistent itching around the affected area (usually in older children, this is where they feel the most pain). If a child complains that their skin itches a lot, then this could be due to an allergic reaction to any insect sting. Older children may also complain of faintness or dizziness.

Cooling Compress

Makes 1 compress. Peppermint's menthol provides a cooling sensation to the skin, while at the same time increasing blood circulation and dispersing the irritants from the bite or sting site.

Ingredients:

- 16 fluid ounces water
- ½ cup dried peppermint leaf
- ¼ cup Epsom salts

Directions:

1. In a small pot with a tight-fitting lid over high heat, combine all the ingredients. Cover and bring to a boil. Remove from the heat.
2. Soak a cloth in the hot tea, holding it in a dry spot and letting it cool in the air until hot but comfortable to the touch.

Bug Bite Relief Spray

Makes 8 fluid ounces (number of applications vary by use). If you regularly walk through clouds of mosquitoes or black flies or live in an area infested with chiggers, you'll want this cooling, itch-relieving spray stocked for when you come inside.

Ingredients:

- 4 fluid ounces nonalcoholic witch hazel extract or apple cider vinegar
- 2 fluid ounces tincture of rose
- 1 fluid ounce tincture of self-heal
- 1 fluid ounce tincture of yarrow

Directions:

1. In a bottle with a fine-mist sprayer top, combine all the ingredients. Cap the bottle and label it.
2. Liberally spray wherever you've been bitten.

Cold and Flu

The cold is generally a disease that causes a runny nose, sore throat, and congestion in the lungs. This cold usually lasts 10 days and can't last more than 2 weeks.

Flu is an illness with fever and muscle aches. The flu also comes with extreme fatigue, cough, headache, body aches, and pains. Just to name a few symptoms of this disease that is highly contagious to others who are not vaccinated against it.

It's difficult to differentiate between the two because they are both respiratory diseases that cause similar symptoms, such as coughs and sneezing. One of the major differences is that colds are caused by viruses, while flu can be caused by bacteria and viruses. There are also different types of colds, such as the stomach flu (not really cold), enterovirus infections (seen in those kids with asthmatic diseases), and airborne infections. (Such as asthma attacks).

The Relevant Tissue States	Heat (inflammatory immune response)
Relevant Herbal Actions	Antiviral, Immune stimulant
Herbal Allies	Elder, Garlic, Pine, Thyme leaf, Yarrow leaf and flower.

Antibiotic treatments don't affect viral respiratory troubles like colds and flu, they only work on bacteria. Herbs, on the other hand, offer effective assistance by supporting the body's innate healing mechanisms.

Colds and flu generally cause very similar symptoms in everyone, but one or another symptom will be most acute for each person.

Elderberry Syrup

Preparation time: 20 minutes.

Cooking time: 2 hours 20 minutes.

Servings: about 1-quart (20 to 60 doses).

Elderberries have an amazing specific capacity to prevent flu viruses from invading the body and replicating themselves; they also fight colds and other viruses. Take this syrup in addition to remedies for your specific symptoms: 1 to 3 tablespoons 3 to 5 times per day whenever you suspect a cold or flu is present.

Ingredients:

- 3 cups fresh elderberries
- 6 cups water
- 1 cinnamon stick or 1 teaspoon powdered cinnamon
- 1 teaspoon powdered ginger
- 1 teaspoon fennel seed
- 1 teaspoon dried chamomile flower
- 2 cups honey, plus more as needed

Directions:

1. In a medium pot over high heat, combine the berries, water, and herbs. Bring to a boil. Reduce the heat and simmer, uncovered, for 1 to 2 hours or until reduced by half.

2. Use a spoon to mash the berries in the pot. Stir, simmer for 15 minutes more, and strain through a wire mesh sieve or cheesecloth. Squeeze the leftover berries well to get out every last bit of fluid.

3. Return the elderberry decoction to the pan and place it over low heat. Add an equal amount of honey, warming it gently as you stir to mix thoroughly with the elderberry decoction.

4. Bottle and label the syrup. It will stay in the refrigerator for several months.

5. **Tip:** Some recipes use sugar, as this creates a shelf-stable product. We try to avoid sugar, so we use honey and keep ours refrigerated. Another alternative is to add 2 cups of tincture (in addition to the decoction and honey) to your syrup the alcohol content will preserve it. Tinctures of ginger, garlic, pine, yarrow, and thyme are all good options.

Constipation

The most common form of constipation is chronic constipation. Chronic means that the person has been having regular bowel movements, but that the stool is still hard and uncomfortable for long periods of time. When someone has been suffering from chronic constipation for more than a few weeks, they are said to be in a state of functional or organic constipation.

Constipation is very common in America: about 40% of adults experience it at least once per year, and many say that they have some sort of discomfort from it on an ongoing basis. It is also a problem in children, and even very young children can develop chronic constipation if they have not seen medical help for their condition.

Constipation can be caused by physical, emotional, or stress-related issues that interfere with normal bowel movements.

Chronic constipation comes with various symptoms that can range from minor problems, such as bloating and low energy, to more severe problems like pain, rectal bleeding, or even the development of hemorrhoids. It is important to see a doctor if you have any symptoms of chronic constipation in order to find out what is causing it.

The Relevant Tissue States	Cold (stagnation), Dryness, Tension
Relevant Herbal Actions	Bitter, Carminative, Demulcent, Hepatic, Laxative
Herbal Allies	Angelica, Dandelion root, Ginger, Marshmallow, Milk thistle seed, St. John's wort leaf and flower

Sometimes, constipation is simply a sign of dehydration—drinks some water! If it's a chronic issue, it may be an indication of a food allergy or simply a sign that you're not getting sufficient fiber in your diet. A good, thick, cold infusion of marshmallow solves both problems: It rehydrates better than water alone, and it includes a lot of polysaccharides and fibers that help move stool along.

Constipation, especially when ongoing, can be traced back to sluggish liver function. Bile produced by the liver is a digestive fluid, but it also lubricates the intestines; when production is low, things can get stuck. Bitters and carminatives help spur digestive function, and liver-restorative herbs (hepatics) such as milk thistle can reestablish normal function.

Bowel-Hydrating Infusion

Preparation time: 10 minutes.

Cooking time: 0 minutes.

Servings: 2(½) cups dried herb mix (enough for 14 to 18 quarts of tea).

A bit tastier than solo marshmallows; this is a great solution for the type of constipation that often afflicts people with dry constitutions. If you have hard-to-pass, dry, little "rabbit pellet" bowel movements, this is for you. Drink a quart or more every day.

Ingredients:

- 1 cup dried linden leaf and flower
- 1 cup dried marshmallow root
- ¼ cup dried cinnamon bark
- ¼ cup dried licorice root

Directions:

1. In a medium bowl, mix all the herbs. Store in an airtight container.
2. Make a cold infusion: Measure 2 to 4 tablespoons of herbs per quart of water and place in a Mason jar or French press. Pour in cold or room-temperature water and steep for 4 to 8 hours before straining.

Bowel-Motivating Tincture

Preparation time: 20 minutes.

Cooking time: 0 minutes.

Servings: 4 fluid ounces (30 to 60 doses)

These bitters and carminatives will spur the bowels to movement by stimulating bile flow and intestinal peristalsis.

Ingredients:

- 1(½) fluid ounces tincture of dandelion root
- ½ fluid ounces tincture of St. John's wort
- ½ fluid ounce tincture of angelica root
- ½ fluid ounce tincture of ginger

Directions:

1. In a small bottle, combine the tinctures. Cap the bottle and label it.

Strains and Sprains

A common injury that's a bit difficult to diagnose is the strain or sprain. A strain is caused by excessive stretching or trauma to a muscle, tendon, or ligament. A sprain is when the joint capsule is overstretched or torn.

Both are injuries that occur when tendons, ligaments, or muscles are stretched or torn. Strains generally happen as the result of overuse or improper use of a muscle, while sprains typically result from injury to the ligament. There is another difference between these two types of injuries—strains and sprains often have different treatments. The most common treatment for a strain is rice. It stands for rest, ice, compression, and elevation—this treatment involves the application of rest, ice therapy over the injury site (which should be kept elevated), compression bandages to reduce swelling and prevent further injury from happening, and finally elevation in order to keep blood flow flowing properly.

If you have pain in your lower leg, for example, that may be due to an overstretched calf muscle. The common treatment for this particular injury would be rice: rest the injured area as much as possible and apply ice after activity. Heat before activity and cold afterward will help offset any inflammation and swelling that might occur in the affected muscles.

A sprain would be more likely to occur in your ankle, knee, or wrist. If the pain is abnormally severe or there is a lot of swelling, be sure to get medical attention promptly.

Fixing sprains and strains normally involves physical therapy, ice, and compression. Your doctor may prescribe anti-inflammatory drugs as well for pain management. Recovery should happen within 4–7 days of treating the injury properly.

Symptomatology	Inflammation
Actions Required	Anti-inflammation, Circulatory stimulant
Recommended Herbs	Ginger root, Solomon's seal root, St. John's wort root, Heal all leaves and flowers, Meadowsweet leaves and flowers, Cinnamon bark, Peppermint leaves, Lizard tail root, Wintergreen leaves, Black Cohosh root, Ashwagandha root, Raspberry root, White Willow bark

Analgesic Tea 1

Preparation time: 10 minutes.

Cooking time: 30 minutes.

Servings : 2

Ingredients:

- 1 teaspoon raspberry root
- 1 teaspoon willow bark
- 1 cup distilled boiling water

Directions:

1. Pour boiling water over the herbs mixture. Let rest for half an hour—strain and drink throughout the day.

Analgesic Tea 2

Preparation time: 5 minutes.

Cooking time: 10 minutes.

Servings : 2

Ingredients:

- 1 teaspoon ashwagandha root
- 1 teaspoon black cohosh root
- 1 cup distilled boiling water

Directions:

1. Pour boiling water over the herbs mixture. Let rest minutes before straining.
2. Drink one cup throughout the day.

Analgesic Ointment

Preparation time: 20 minutes.

Cooking time: 2 hours.

Servings : 2

Ingredients:

- 2 tablespoons wintergreen leaves tincture
- 3 tablespoons lizard tail root tincture
- 1 pound coconut oil

Directions:

1. Melt the coconut oil in a water bath. Add the herbs, stir and let on low heat for two hours. Strain and pour in a mason jar, let it cool down, and then close the lid.
2. Apply on the sore part whenever needed and massage.

Sprain Healing Ointment

Preparation time: 10 minutes.

Cooking time: 30 minutes.

Servings : 2

Ingredients:

- 1 tablespoon ashwagandha root oil
- 1 tablespoon St. John's wort root oil
- 1 tablespoon Solomon's seal root oil
- 1 tablespoon heal all leaves and flowers oil
- 1 tablespoon meadowsweet root oil

Directions:

1. Combine the essential oils in the proportion indicated above. Place 10 drops on your hands, rub vigorously to warm up the oil, and massage the sore part.

Conclusion

Healing plants were used by the Indians of North America long before the arrival of Europeans. The use of natural remedies can be traced to the medicine men, who, through their intimate contact with nature, became great healers and experts in herbal medicine.

The American Indians had learned that certain plants had healing powers for their ills, and they found it easy to identify these plants in the forest where they lived. They also discovered that certain plant roots would cure headaches or asthma if they boiled them in water until only a small amount was left. Other herbs, which cured a cough, could be made into syrup by boiling them with sugar to make cough medicine.

If an American Indian was sick, they asked their medicine man to choose the right plant for them. In selecting a plant, the medicine man had to consider what part of nature it represented — its appearance, smell, and taste were all important factors in the selection. The medicine man also chose a plant that would improve the condition of particular parts of the body and one which would have a beneficial effect on the mind.

After finding out about their symptoms and requirements, these people traveled for miles into the forest, searching for plants to cure them. They used several methods to find plants; for example, one method was to call out the name of a plant and listen for its response, and another method was to look for pieces of plants that bore the most desirable fruits or seeds and then to examine them.

Often, the medicine man would find a fruit or root which looked as though it had been bitten by some animal. When he pushed the fruit or root aside with his hand, another plant would grow out of the stump so that they were plants that bore fruit down below instead of on top of the trees, like other plants.

Part XI

~

Native American At Home - Do It Yourself

Most Common DIY Herbal Recipes

Herbal teas differ widely from one another, and the general teas because they do not come from the same plant. They are the combinations of flowers, herbs, and dried fruits — which are brewed like tea. Herbal teas contain no caffeine, often lower blood pressure, have delicious flavors, and improve digestion. They also often contain no calories and no sugar.

Raspberry Tea

Servings: 1

Brewing Time: 10 minutes

Ingredients:

- 1 cup water
- ¼ cup dried raspberry leaves
- ¼ cup dried lemongrass
- ½ cup dried chamomile flowers
- ½ cup dried orange peel

Directions:

1. Mix all the dried herbs listed above.
2. Boil the water.
3. Add 1 teaspoon of the tea mixture to a cup.
4. Pour the hot water over it. Cover and steep for 5–10 minutes.
5. The longer the time, the more tannin is extracted.
6. Consume hot, cold, or iced.

Hibiscus-Ginger Tea

Servings: 4

Brewing Time: 15 minutes

Ingredients:

- 4 cups water
- 1 tbsp. hibiscus leaves
- 1 tbsp. grated fresh ginger
- 3–5 mint leaves

Directions:

1. Boil the water in a pot.
2. Take the hibiscus and ginger and blend them in another pot.
3. Pour the hot water over the tea mixture, cover, and steep for 10–12 minutes.

4. The color of the tea will turn ruby red, then add the mint leaves for a fresh flavor.
5. Serve hot or cold.

Mint Tea

Servings: 2

Brewing Time: 8 minutes

Ingredients:

- 2 cups water
- 15–20 fresh mint leaves
- 2 lemon slices
- 1 tsp. honey (optional)

Directions:

1. In a teapot, boil the water.
2. Remove from the heat and add in all the mint leaves. Cover the pot and steep for 5 minutes. Increase the time for a strong flavor of mint.
3. Pour it into a cup or glass.
4. Add the honey and garnish with the lemon slices.
5. Enjoy hot or iced.

Sweet and Spicy Herb Tea

Servings: 1

Brewing Time: 10 minutes

Ingredients:

- 1 cup water
- ½ tbsp. cloves
- 1 tbsp. dried stevia
- ¼ cup cinnamon sticks
- ¼ cup dried orange zest
- ¼ cup dried chamomile flowers
- ½ cup dried lemon verbena

Directions:

1. Make the blend and use 1 teaspoon of the tea mixture.
2. Boil the water and pour it over the tea mixture.
3. Cover the pot and let it steep for 5 minutes or more.
4. Strain it into a cup and serve it hot. Alternatively, pour it over ice in a glass and serve cold.
5. Enjoy the sweet and spicy taste.

Basil Tea

Servings: 1

Brewing Time: 5 minutes

Ingredients:

- 1 cup water
- 1 tsp. basil leaves
- ¼ tsp. dried ginger
- ½ tsp. cinnamon powder
- 1 tsp. honey (optional)

Directions:

1. Boil the water and add the basil leaves, ginger, and cinnamon.
2. Steep it for 5 minutes.
3. Strain it and add the honey to improve the taste.
4. Pour it in a cup and serve hot.

Lavender Tea

Ingredients:

- 2 cups water
- 5 tbsp. lemon balm
- 2 tbsp. dried lavender flower
- 1 tbsp. honey

Directions:

1. Boil the water in a pot.
2. Add all the ingredients to the serving cup and mix well.
3. Pour the boiling water into a serving cup with the lemon balm mixture.
4. Cover the cup and steep it for 8 minutes. (You can mix in honey as per your taste.)
5. Strain the tea.

6. Serve and enjoy it.

Mint Tea

Ingredients:

- 2 tbsp. rosemary
- 3 tbsp. mint
- Water

Directions:

1. Add the water to the pot and bring it to a boil.
2. Add the rosemary and cover the pot for few minutes.
3. Add the mint leaves to the cup and pour the boiling rosemary water over it.
4. Cover the cup and let it steep for few minutes. (You can add lemon juice to enhance the taste.)
5. Serve and enjoy it.

Lemon and Elderflower Tea

Ingredients:

- 1 tsp. honey
- 1 tbsp. elderflower
- 1 tsp. lime juice

Directions:

1. Boil the water in a pot.
2. Add all the ingredients and mix well.
3. Cover the pot and let it boil over low heat for 15 minutes.
4. Strain the tea in a serving cup.
5. Serve and enjoy it.

Chamomile and lemon balm

Ingredients:

- ⅓ tbsp. dried chamomile
- ⅓ tbsp. lemon balm leaves, crushed and dried

Directions:

1. Boil the water in a pot.
2. Add all the ingredients and mix well.
3. Cover the pot and let it boil for 15 minutes over low heat.
4. Strain the tea in a serving cup.
5. Serve and enjoy it.

Decoctions

A decoction is a concentrated liquid obtained from boiling or heating a material. The word decoction is commonly used for a medicinal extract attained from the herbal plant's heating bark, stem, or roots. A decoction is different from an infusion in that the part of the plant used to obtain them, i.e., to gain infusion, the leaves or flower of the plant, is used while collecting decoction bark, or root of the plant is used.

American Liver Cleansing Tonic

Ingredients:

- ⅓ tsp. sassafras
- ⅓ tsp. ginger
- ⅓ tsp. dandelion
- Water

Directions:

1. Add the water to a pot and stir in the ingredients.
2. Bring it to a boil.
3. Reduce the heat to low and cover the pot.
4. Let it cook for 20 minutes.
5. Remove the pot from the heat and keep it aside for 5 minutes while the lid is over the pot. (You may stir in honey if needed.)
6. Serve and enjoy it.

Bronchitis Soother

Ingredients:

- ⅓ tsp. colt foot
- ⅓ tsp. marshmallow
- ⅓ tsp. comfrey
- ⅓ tsp. mullein
- Water

Directions:

1. Add the water to a pot and mix in all the ingredients. Keep it aside for 20 minutes.
2. Place the pot over medium heat and let it boil.
3. Cover the pot and reduce the heat to low.

4. Let it cook for 20 minutes. (You may add honey according to your taste.)
5. Serve and enjoy it.

Note: This tea is best to get relief from asthma, sore throat, cough, bronchitis, and most respiratory system issues.

Chaga Mushroom Coffee

Ingredients:

- 2 tbsp. chaga
- 1 ⅓ cups water

Directions:

1. Add the chaga in water in a pot.
2. Place the pot over medium heat and let it boil.
3. Cover the pot and let it simmer for 15 minutes. (You may mix in honey according to your taste.)
4. Serve and enjoy it.

Note: This coffee acts as a stimulator for your immune system and prevents cancer development.

Echinacea Decoction

Ingredients:

- 1 tbsp. Echinacea
- 1 ½ cups water

Directions:

1. Add the water to a pot and add the Echinacea root to it.
2. Place the pot over medium heat and bring it to a boil.
3. Cover the pot and let it simmer for 35 minutes over low heat.

4. Transfer the decoction to the serving cup using the filter to remove the herb.
5. Serve and enjoy it.

Note: This decoction will boost your immune system and will help you to fight various diseases.

Hawthorn Berry Syrup

Ingredients:

- 1 ½ cups water
- 1 tbsp. hawthorn berry, crushed

Directions:

8.

1. Combine the hawthorn and water in a pot.
2. Place the pot over medium heat and let it boil.
3. Cover the pot and reduce the heat.
4. Let it simmer for 20 minutes.
5. Strain the syrup and preserve it for later use.
6. Use 1 tablespoon of hawthorn syrup with honey in warm water and drink it once a day.
7. This decoction is best for cardiovascular diseases.

Popsicles

Fruit Popsicles with Coconut

Ingredients:

- 3 cups coconut water
- 5 kiwi slices
- ½ cup black grapes
- ½ cup strawberry, sliced
- ½ cup pineapple

Directions:

1. Combine all the fruits in a container.
2. Transfer the fruit mixture to the mold.
3. Fill the mold with coconut water.
4. Cover the mold and put it in the freezer for a few hours.
5. Serve and enjoy it.

Watermelon Mint Popsicles

Ingredients:

- 5 cups sliced watermelon
- ⅓ cup chopped mint
- ½ cup lime juice

Directions:

1. Add all the ingredients to the food processor and blend to get a smooth purée.
2. Strain the purée in a bowl.
3. Transfer the purée into the mold and put it in the freezer for a few hours.
4. Serve and enjoy it.

Cucumber Mint Popsicles

Ingredients:

- ⅓ cup lime juice
- ½ cup chopped mint leaves
- 2 cups chopped cucumber
- 2 cups water
- ⅓ cup sugar
- 1 tsp. green tea powder

Directions:

1. Add the water to the pot and let it boil.
2. Stir in the sugar and reduce the heat to low.
3. Let the sugar dissolve to get syrup.

4. Mix in the mint and stir well. Cook for a few minutes to give syrup the flavor of mint.
5. Remove the pot from the heat and set it aside.
6. Remove the mint leaves from the syrup.
7. Place the mint syrup in the fridge for a few minutes.
8. Add all the remaining ingredients to the blender and blend them to get a smooth purée.
9. Add the mint syrup slowly to adjust the taste.
10. Transfer the purée into a mold and place it in the freezer for a few hours.
11. Serve and enjoy it.

Mint Lemon Popsicles

Ingredients:

- 1 tbsp. lime peel
- 2 tbsp. lemon juice
- 3 cups water
- 3 tsp. honey
- 1 cup mint leaves

Directions:

1. Add the water to a pot and bring it to a boil.
2. Mix in all the remaining ingredients and cook for a few minutes to fully mix them.
3. Remove the pot from the heat and let it stand for a while.
4. Transfer the mixture to the mold and place it in the freezer for a few hours.
5. Serve and enjoy it.

Pine Popsicles

Ingredients:

- ½ cup pine needles
- 3 cups water
- 3 lemon slices
- 1 clove, crushed
- 1 tbsp. ginger
- 1 tsp. green tea
- 2 tbsp. lemon juice
- ½ cup jaggery

Directions:

1. Add the water to the pot and bring it to a boil.
2. Mix in the pine needles, clove, and ginger. Cook for a few minutes.
3. Now stir in the jaggery and let it boil for 5 minutes.
4. Mix in the green tea and stir well.
5. Reduce the heat to low and cover the pot. Let it steep for 5 minutes.
6. Add the lemon slices, remove the pot from the heat, and let it stand for a while.
7. Strain the mixture in cups and set aside.
8. Place the cups in the freezer and freeze them for 80 minutes.
9. Serve and enjoy it.

Strawberry Basil Popsicles

Ingredients:

- 1 cup sliced strawberries
- 1 tbsp. lemon zest
- ½ cup sugar syrup
- 1 ½ cups basil leaves
- ¼ cup Tofutti® cream

Directions:

1. Add lemon zest, ½ cup of basil leaves, strawberries, and syrup to the food processor. Blend to get a purée.
2. Transfer the strawberry purée into a mold and place it in the freezer for 2 hours.
3. Add the cream, remaining basil, and syrup into the blender. Blend to get a smooth purée.
4. Remove the strawberry mold from the freezer and pour the bail purée over it.
5. Place the mold again in the freezer and freeze for a few hours.
6. Serve and enjoy it.

Lavender Moon Milk Popsicles

Ingredients:

- 1 cup coconut cream
- ½ tsp. ashwagandha powder
- 2 tbsp. lavender
- 1 ½ tbsp. honey
- 1 vanilla bean

- Water

Directions:

1. Add the cream to a bowl and whisk until fluffy.
2. Add the water and beat again to get 2 cups.
3. Place the bowl over medium heat.
4. Add the vanilla beans and lavender and mix well. Cook for 5 minutes.
5. Remove the pot from the heat and set it aside.
6. Strain the mixture.
7. Add the honey and ashwagandha, and toss well.
8. Place the mixture in the fridge for 30 minutes.
9. Transfer the mixture into a mold, and then place it in the freezer.
10. Freeze for a few hours. Serve and enjoy it.

Lemon Verbena Sun Tea Popsicles

Ingredients:

- 2 cups water
- 1 cup pineapple juice
- 2 tbsp. verbena

Directions:

1. Add verbena and water in a jar. Cover the jar and shake well.
2. Place the jar in the sunshine for a few hours to extract the essence of the herb.
3. Strain the mixture and set it aside.
4. Add the pineapple juice to the mixture and toss well.
5. Transfer the mixture into a mold, place the mold in the freezer, and freeze it for few hours.
6. Serve and enjoy it.

Basil and Aloe Vera Ice Cubes

Ingredients:

- 1 cups basil
- 2 tbsp. Aloe Vera gel mixture

Directions:

1. Add the basil leaves into the blender with water, and blend to get a smooth mixture.
2. Add the Aloe Vera gel and toss well.

3. Transfer the mixture to an ice cube tray, then place it in the freezer.
4. Freeze for a few hours.

Mint Ice Cubes

Ingredients:

- Mint leaves
- Water

Directions:

1. Add the mint leaves to an ice cube tray, and then pour in water to fill the tray part.
2. Place the tray in the freezer, and freeze.

Ginger and Garlic Ice Cubes

Ingredients:

- 1 cup garlic
- 1 cup ginger

Directions:

1. Add the garlic and ginger to a food processor and blend to get a paste.
2. Transfer the paste to an ice cube tray and place it in the freezer.
3. Freeze for a few hours.

Lime Ice Cubes

Ingredients:

- Lemon juice

Directions:

1. Add the lemon juice to an ice cube tray and freeze it for several hours.

Coffee Ice Cubes

Ingredients:

- 4 tbsp. coffee
- 2 cups water

Directions:

1. Add the water to the pot and bring it to a boil.
2. Mix in coffee and stir well.
3. Cook for a few minutes.
4. Remove the pot from the heat and let it stand for few hours.
5. Transfer the coffee solution into an ice cube tray, and freeze it for a few hours.

Masala Tea Ice Cubes

Ingredients:

- 1 ½ cups water
- 1 star anise
- 1 cardamom stick
- 3 cloves
- 2 tbsp. ginger
- 1 tbsp. black pepper
- ½ cup milk
- 4 tbsp. black tea leaves
- 1 tbsp. sugar

Directions:

1. Add the water to a pan and bring it to a boil.
2. Mix in all the spices and cook for 15 minutes.
3. Stir in the milk and reduce the heat to low.
4. Cover the pan and simmer it for 5 minutes.
5. Add the black tea leaves and mix well. Cook for another 5 minutes.
6. Strain the tea and let it stand for a few minutes. Transfer the tea into an ice cubes tray and then freeze it.

Cucumber and Lemon Ice Cubes

Ingredients:

- 1 cup cucumber
- 4 tbsp. lemon juice

Directions:

1. Add the cucumber and lemon juice into a blender and blend to get a purée.
2. Transfer the purée into an ice cube tray and freeze it for several hours.

Berry Cubes

Ingredients:

- Berries (strawberry, blackberry, and blueberry)
- Water

Directions:

1. Add the berries to an ice cube tray and add the water.
2. Place the tray in the freezer, and freeze for a few hours.

Hot Chocolate Ice Cubes

Ingredients:

- 3 tbsp. cocoa powder
- 1 tsp. vanilla essence

- 2 cups milk

Directions:

1. Add the milk to a pan and boil it.
2. Add the cocoa powder and vanilla, and stir well.
3. Cook for a few minutes to completely dissolve everything well.
4. Transfer the mixture to an ice cube tray, and freeze it.

Baths

Relaxing Herbal Foot Bath

Ingredients:

- ½ cup lavender
- 1 cup sage
- ½ cup hops
- ¼ cup rosemary
- Water

Directions:

1. Add the water to a pan and let it boil.
2. Add the herbs and stir well.
3. Cover the pan and reduce the heat.
4. Let it simmer for 15 minutes.
5. Transfer the mixture basin and add the water.
6. Cover the basin with a sheet to contain the loss of heat.
7. Dip your feet and relax for 25 minutes.

Herbal Face Steam

Ingredients:

- 1 tbsp. thyme
- 1 tbsp. lavender
- 1 tbsp. basil
- 1 tbsp. eucalyptus
- 1 tbsp. rosemary
- 1 tbsp. peppermint
- 1 tbsp. oregano
- Water

Directions:

1. Boil the water in the pot over medium heat.
2. Add the herbs to a wide-mouthed pot, and pour in the boiling water.
3. Mix well, cover the pot with the lid, and leave for 3 minutes.
4. Before leaning over the pot to get steam, check the temperature not to burn your skin.
5. Lean over the pot and slowly inhale and exhale for about 10 minutes.

Herbal Bath Salts

Ingredients:

- 3 cups salt, Epsom and Himalayan pink
- ½ cup baking soda
- 3 tbsp. olive oil
- ½ cup dried rose petals
- 6 tsp. lavender oil
- 6 tsp. rosemary oil
- ½ cup dried lavender flower
- 8 tsp. cardamom oil
- ½ cup dried basil

Directions:

1. Combine all the ingredients in a food processor and blend to get a paste.
2. Transfer the paste into the jar and store it for later use.
3. Add 4 tablespoons of the paste into the bathing water and stir well.
4. Enjoy your relaxing and medicating bath.

Anti-Inflammatory Bath Tea

Ingredients:

- ½ cup ginger
- 5 cups water
- ½ cup dried birch bark
- 2 cups Epsom salt
- ½ cup dried yarrow

Directions:

1. Add the water to a pot over medium heat.
2. Add the bark and ginger, and stir well.
3. Let it boil, and then reduce the heat to low and cover the pot.
4. Cook for 15 minutes.
5. Mix in the yarrow and cook for another 10 minutes.
6. Strain the mixture until the anti-inflammatory bath tea is ready.
7. Add the mixture into the bathing tub and enjoy your bath.

Cold Herbal Compresses

Ingredients:

- 1 green tea bag
- 1 peppermint tea bag
- 1 chamomile-lavender tea bag
- 1 cup water
- Eucalyptus essential oil
- Lavender essential oil

Directions:

1. Add the water to a pot and let it boil.
2. Add tea bags into a cup.
3. Pour into the boiling water and cover the cup.
4. Let it steep for 25 minutes.
5. Soak a towel or washcloth into the tea solution and leave it there for a few minutes.
6. Squeeze gently to remove any extra liquid.
7. The washcloth should be wet but without liquid dripping.
8. Now drizzle 1 tablespoon of eucalyptus essential oil over the wet washcloth.
9. Apply this medicated washcloth around your feet, chest, and anywhere you want.

Note: This herbal compresses remedy will help you relax during summer, give smoothness to your eyes, and may also enhance the glow of your skin.

Hot Herbal Pouch

Ingredients:

- 2 tbsp. ginger
- 10 eucalyptus leaves
- 5 tbsp. lime peel
- 2 tbsp. lemongrass
- 1 tbsp. tamarind powder
- 2 tsp. salt
- 3 tsp. camphor granules

Directions:

1. Combine all the ingredients in a bowl.
2. Transfer the mixture to a washcloth, make a pouch, and tie it.
3. Place the pouch in hot water and massage the targeted area.

Laotian Herbal Compress

Ingredients:

- 8 tbsp. cooked rice
- 2 tbsp. basil
- 3 tbsp. lemongrass
- 3 tbsp. peppermint
- 2 tbsp. ginger
- 4 tbsp. cinnamon

Directions:

1. Combine all the ingredients in a bowl.
2. Transfer the mixture to a washcloth, make a pouch, and tie it.
3. Place the pouch in hot water and massage the targeted area.

Chamomile Cold Compress

Ingredients:

- 4 cups hot water
- 2 tsp. chamomile tea

Directions:

1. Add the water to a pan and mix in the chamomile tea.
2. Cover the pan and let it steep for a few minutes.
3. Let it stand for a while to cool it down.
4. Soak the washcloth into the tea mixture and squeeze the extra liquid.
5. Place the washcloth over the targeted area for more than 10 minutes and experience the effect.

Bali Herbal Compress Ball

Ingredients:

- 3 tbsp. ginger
- 3 cloves
- 5 tbsp. rice powder
- 1 tbsp. turmeric powder
- 1 tbsp. coriander
- 1 tbsp. cinnamon
- Water

Directions:

1. Combine all the ingredients in a bowl and toss well to mix everything.
2. Transfer the mixture to a washcloth and fold to make a ball.
3. Tie the cloth with the yarn.
4. Add the water to a pan and bring it to a boil.
5. Place the herbal compress in the boiling water for 30 minutes.
6. Remove the ball from the water and let it stand for a while. When the temperature is bearable, use it in the targeted area.

Herbal Healing Salve

Ingredients:

- ½ cup calendula almond oil
- ⅓ cup beeswax
- ½ cup comfrey almond oil
- ½ tsp. essential oil of rose geranium
- ½ cup plantain infused almond oil
- 8 tbsp. herbal mixture
- Water

Directions:

1. Add the herbal mixture into a jar and pour over the almond oil.
2. Close the lid and shake well.
3. Place the jar in a warm place for more than 65 days.
4. Strain the oil from the mixture using cheesecloth and discard the solids content of the mixture.
5. Store at the dim place. Then the infused oil for the salve is ready.
6. Now add the water to a pot and let it boil.
7. Add the beeswax to a small pan and place the pan over the boiling water to melt the wax.
8. When the wax is melted, add the infused oils to it, and stir well.
9. Remove the pan from the boiling water and set it aside for a while. (It will take few hours to cool down.) The healing salve is ready to use.

Herbal Poultice

Ingredients:

- 1 tsp. turmeric powder
- 2 tsp. coconut oil
- ¼ cup sliced onion
- 1 tsp. garlic
- 4 tbsp. ginger paste

Directions:

1. Combine all the ingredients in a pan and cook over low heat until the content gets dry.
2. Remove the pan from the heat and let it stand for a while.
3. Transfer the mixture into the cheesecloth, then fold the cloth and tie it.

4. Message the affected area with the pouch for about 30 minutes. (This poultice is used as an anti-inflammatory agent.)

Bran Poultice

Ingredients:

- Water
- Bran

Directions:

1. Add the water to a pot and boil it.
2. Add the bran and mix well to form a paste.
3. Apply while hot on the affected area. (This poultice can be used to relieve strains, bruises, and inflammation.)

Mustard Poultice

Ingredients:

- Mustard powder
- Water
- Flour

Directions:

4. Add the mustard powder to the water and make a paste.
5. Use the flour to thicken the paste.
6. Add in a cloth and message. (It can be used to treat arthritis and to improve circulation.)

Bread Poultice

Ingredients:

- Bread, sliced
- Milk

Directions:

1. Add the milk to a pot and heat it over medium heat.
2. Keep it aside to cool down a little.
3. Add the bread slices and let them stand in the warm milk.
4. Mix the bread with the milk to form a paste.
5. Now apply it over the skin and leave it for about 20 minutes. (You can use it on a cyst, splinter, and abscess.)

Potato poultices

Ingredients:

- Grated potato
- Water

Directions:

1. Add the water to a pan and boil it.
2. Add the grated potato and make a paste.
3. Apply over the inflamed area for 10 minutes. (It can be used as a pain reliever and provides a cooling effect. Apply on carbuncles and boils.)

Washcloths

Washcloths are used to gently clean the baby's face, lips, eyes, and genitals. They can be used in the bath area as well. They can be used on a critically ill patient who cannot survive an active bath. In this comfortable way, medicine can easily be applied to the skin, and thus it can be transferred to a deeper area of the body through diffusion.

Washcloths can be warm by using hot infusions of medicine when specific impacts of heating are needed, or they can be cold when benefits of cold are needed. It all depends upon personal choice as well as symptoms of illnesses. For acute injuries, for example, brushing and combat sports fights, cold washcloths with specific benefits of ice and anti-inflammatory medicine can be a smart choice to limit swelling and bruising as well as impeding bleeding from fresh wounds.

When used cold, they have anesthetic properties, which make them a natural painkiller. When used warm, washcloths can stimulate blood flow due to vasodilator effects, as well as a soothing response of the body can also be obtained.

Herbal washcloths can be applied to the area of an injury. Here are different ways to make herbal washcloths to be used for different conditions.

Eye Wash

Ingredients:

- Water
- Peppermint essential oil

Directions:

1. Add a few drops of water into an eye spray bottle.
2. Fill the rest of the bottle with peppermint essential oil.
3. Use these eye drops to clean the eye area.

Note: This is very good for people who suffer from dry eyes, as they can treat them with one quick and simple treatment. Refrigerate it in an air-tight container after each use to ensure potency. Eyewashes can also be used for other purposes as well, such as treating conjunctivitis, blepharitis, and other eye issues.

Tongue Wash

Ingredients:

- Water
- Thyme essential oil

Directions:

1. Add a few drops of water to the tongue spray bottle.
2. Fill the rest of the bottle with thyme essential oil.
3. Use this tongue spray to clean the area around the mouth, and with this, you would feel a soothing sensation on your tongue.

Note: This is a very good treatment if your mouth is filled with bad breath and as well as a cleansing of the inside of your mouth. It can be stored for two weeks in an air-tight container after use. Tongue washes can be used on other parts of the body, such as the inner thigh area, groin area, armpit, and any other areas that may need a light cleaning along with soothing.

Armpit Wash

Ingredients:

- Water
- Lavender essential oil

Directions:

1. Add a few drops of water to the armpit spray bottle.
2. Fill the rest of the bottle with lavender essential oil.
3. Use this armpit spray to clean your armpits, and you will feel a soothing sensation on your skin.

Note: This is very good for people who work in the construction field, as it will help remove odors from the body and develop an anti-bacterial treatment for skin infections. It can be stored for two weeks in an air-tight container after use.

The armpit wash can also be used on other areas of the body, such as a groin area, inner thigh area, and back of the neck, to get a good cleaning.

Inner Thigh Wash

Ingredients:

- Water
- Lavender essential oil

Directions:

1. Add a few drops of water to the inner thigh spray bottle.
2. Fill the rest of the bottle with lavender essential oil.
3. Use this inner thigh spray to clean the area around your groin, and it will make you feel a soothing sensation.

Note: This is very good for people who play sports, as it will help in removing perspiration and bacteria that may cause infections. It can create an anti-bacterial treatment for skin infections. It can be stored for two weeks in an air-tight container after use.

The inner thigh wash can be used in other areas, such as the armpit, groin, inner wrist, and any other not-to-be-replaced areas.

Inner Wrist Wash

Ingredients:

- Water
- Lavender essential oil

Preparation:

1. Add a few drops of water to the inner wrist spray bottle.
2. Fill the rest of the bottle with lavender essential oil.

3. Use this inner wrist spray to clean the area around your hand, and it will make you feel a soothing sensation.

Note: The inner wrist wash can also be used in other areas of the body, such as the groin area, armpit, inner thigh area, or any other not-to-be-replaced areas.

Differences Between Compresses and a Washcloth

Compresses are usually smaller and thicker than standard washcloths. They also tend to be softer due to the materials that they are made out of. Compresses are generally used in larger areas compared to a washcloth, with compresses being made for specific parts of the body like the head, neck, back, or stomach.

Washcloths can be used for a multitude of jobs, but their biggest use is for cleaning the skin. They can also work as an extra towel, but they should never be mixed with another laundry because it could lead to mold buildup on one or both items.

Washcloths are typically much smaller than a regular towel, but they should also be used for specific parts of the body. Washcloths should not be used for drying or cleaning your hair or face.

Compresses and washcloths can either be made out of cotton gauze, flannel, or linen. Linen is extremely soft and durable, while flannel is extremely soft and absorbent.

Cotton gauze and flannel can easily become damaged if used excessively, which could lead to germs getting passed on, along with some discomfort in the skin. Cotton gauze is known to cause a burning sensation when being used in certain parts of the body, especially when people have sensitive skin or allergies. Linen is not only the softest material used to make compresses, but it is also very durable.

For cleaning, washcloths can be thrown directly in the washer with the rest of your laundry load. Compresses are a little more delicate and should be hand-washed instead of thrown in a washer. If you do decide to throw your compresses in the washer, you should separate them from other items. You will also want to use cold water when washing your compresses, as hot water can shrink or damage their shape.

Herbal Recipes for Personal Hygiene, Home Purification, and Pet Care

This chapter will offer you an overview of the various herbal recipes and strategies for personal cleanliness, pet care, and home purification.

Athletes Foot

It's a disorder that usually affects athletes because their feet sweat a lot, but it can also affect non-athletes if their feet sweat a lot too. Itching and rashes under the foot are among the symptoms.

A Poultice Containing Garlic for Athlete Foot

Ingredients:

- 1 tsp. honey
- 2 tsp. fresh garlic

Directions:

1. Add both garlic and honey to a mixing bowl.
2. Dip a cotton swab in the poultice and gently rub it on your foot.
3. In just a few days, you'll get extraordinary results.

Gingivitis

Gingivitis is the inflammation of the gums that happens when a person does not maintain proper oral hygiene. It can be excruciatingly painful, and in difficult situations, the tooth may fall loose.

Mouthwash Containing Chamomile and Calendula for Gingivitis

Ingredients:

- 1 oz. chamomile, dry form
- 4 cups water
- 1 oz. calendula, dry form

Directions:

1. In a pan, combine all the ingredients and heat until the liquid has reduced by half.
2. Strain the mixture through a cheesecloth and discard the herbs.
3. Put the mouthwash in a sterile jar and keep it there.

4. Apply two tbsp. to your gums twice a day and see the results; you'll be able to get rid of your sore gums in no time.

Tooth Decay

It happens when the enamel on the surface of the tooth softens, and the tooth turns black. As the tooth begins to expose the capillaries, it can be extremely painful, and as a result, eating becomes the most painful task.

Peppermint and Sage for Tooth Decay

Ingredients:

- 1 oz. peppermint, dry form
- 4 cups water
- 1 oz. sage, dry form

Directions:

1. In a pan, combine all the ingredients and heat until the liquid has reduced by half.
2. Strain the mixture through a cheesecloth and discard the herbs.
3. Put the mouthwash in a sterile jar and keep it there.
4. Use 2 tsp. every day and check the results; you'll be free of tooth decay in no time.

Essential Oil Mixture for Head Lice

Ingredients:

- 1 oz. peppermint, dry form
- 4 drops Neem® essential oil
- ½ cup coconut oil

Directions:

1. Combine all the ingredients in a large mixing bowl and heat the mixture for a few minutes.
2. Apply the oil to your hair and see the results; your lice will be gone in no time.

Note: Tea Tree oil can be replaced with peppermint or eucalyptus essential oils.

Herbal Recipes to Purify Home

The purification of a home is a priority for every single person. However, as noted below, numerous concerns frequently develop in our homes and must be addressed.

Mold production on the Ceiling

Mold growth can be a problem, especially when the rainy season begins because mold growth begins quickly, and our ceilings and walls can be a hotspot for this unpleasant growth.

Garlic and Thyme Compress to Prevent Mold Growth on Walls and Ceilings

Ingredients:

- 1 cup water
- 2 tsp. dried thyme

- 2 tsp. fresh garlic

Directions:

1. Fill a pan halfway with the water and bring it to a boil.
2. Add the garlic and thyme and cook for a few minutes, covered.
3. Strain the infused water into a mug using a cheesecloth.
4. Clean the moldy spots with a cotton swab dipped in the compress for fifteen minutes. Within a few days, you will notice extraordinary results.

Keeping Lizards Away

Lizards and other wall-crawling insects can be unsanitary and even frightening to some people. But, following this excellent natural recipe, you may not need to use synthetic products to keep them away any longer.

Keeping Lizards Away from Your Home with Black Pepper and Coffee Bzalls

Ingredients:

- 1 tsp. coffee
- 1 tbsp. black pepper
- Water, as needed

Directions:

1. You can combine all the ingredients to form round ball structures.
2. Store these balls in a netted pouch in various parts of the house. Lizards will no longer be a resident of your home.

Mosquitoes in the House

Mosquitoes are common in homes and can be quite dangerous since they spread malaria. To get rid of them, use the herbal remedies listed below:

Lavender and Lemongrass Candles for Mosquito Repellent in the Home

Ingredients:

- 1 tsp. lemongrass essential oil
- 1 tsp. lavender essential oil
- 1 cup candle wax

Directions:

1. In a double boiler, combine all the ingredients.
2. Remove the mixture from the bowl and place it in a dark-colored jar with a thread for lighting the candle.
3. Now, every day, light this candle to keep your home mosquito-free.

Killing Bugs

Bugs can become a big part of your home, and different bugs can irritate you a lot. To get rid of these bugs, use the recipes below:

Bug Spray with Witch Hazel, Peppermint, Spearmint, Lavender, and Lemongrass

Ingredients:

- 20 drops lavender essential oil
- 1 tbsp. natural vodka
- ½ cup vinegar
- 1 tbsp. lemongrass
- 1 cup water
- ½ cup rubbing alcohol or witch hazel
- 20 drops peppermint essential oil
- 20 drops spearmint essential oil

Directions:

1. Combine all the ingredients in a mixing bowl.
2. Pour the mixture into a dark spray bottle with a spray head.
3. Spray the mixture around your home to keep it fresh, fragrant, and bug-free.

Herbal Recipes for Pet Care

Pet care is essential since pets are an integral part of our lives. Our dogs have a variety of issues, which can be treated naturally by following herbal recipes.

Treatment for Fleas

Ticks and fleas are most commonly seen in cats and dogs, and they can be treated by bathing them in the following solution:

Flea Treatment with a Body Bath

Ingredients:

- 40 drops rosemary extracts, essential oil
- 40 drops sage extracts, essential oil
- 1 cup unaromatic herbal conditioner

Directions:

1. In a large mixing basin, combine the solution and the basic oil, stirring thoroughly with a whisk or a beater.
2. Transfer it to a plastic jug with a pressing top using a pipe.
3. While washing your pet, add a small amount of the body bath to your pet's body, changing the amount used to cover it completely.
4. Wait for 2 to 5 minutes before washing away the body bath with cold water. Increase your use of it for better results.

Diarrhea

Diarrhea is common in pets, and it can be readily treated by following the recipe below:

Catnip and Sienna Tea for Diarrhea in Pets

Ingredients:

- 1 oz. dried senna leaves
- 1 cup water
- 1 tsp. dried catnip
- 1 tbsp. honey

Directions:

1. Bring the water to a boil and pour it into a cup.
2. Place all the herbs in the cup and cover it with a lid for a few minutes.
3. After a while, strain the tea and add the honey when the herbs have beautifully mingled in the water.
4. Drink this tea 3 to 4 times a day, and your pet's ailment will be solved.

Animal Injuries

Our pets are prone to getting bruises and injuries from time to time. The following solution is simple to use in treating this condition.

Hyssop Poultice for Pet Injuries

Ingredients:

- 2 tsp. fresh hyssop leaves

Directions:

1. Apply the fresh hyssop leaves to the injury and massage for 15 minutes.
2. In just a few days, you'll get extraordinary results.

Coughing in Animals

Cough is also fairly prevalent in many pets, and the following recipes can readily cure it.

Elecampane Root Tea for Cough in Dogs and Cats

Ingredients:

- 1 cup water
- 1 tsp. dried elecampane root
- 1 tbsp. honey

Directions:

1. Bring the water to a boil and pour it into a cup.
2. Place all the herbs in the cup and cover it with a lid for a few minutes.
3. After a while, strain the tea and add honey when the herbs have beautifully mingled in the water.
4. If you give this tea to your pet 3 to 4 times a day, it will cure their cough.

All the recipes shown above are quite helpful and can be utilized for a variety of purposes.

Part XII

~

How to Become an Expert Herbalist

Handling Herbal Medicine

Herbal medicine can be very effective and safe; however, it's also important to understand and respect some safety warnings when using herbal remedies.

In this chapter, we'll talk about some of the best ways to use herbal medicine and why it's important to follow specific recipes and guidelines.

Best Practices and Safety

It's important to follow these practices to keep herbal medicine safe and effective:

- **Know the difference between internal and external medicine:** Herbal remedies have precise uses. You need to know whether the remedy you want to use is for internal or external use. Taking an external remedy internally can cause a lot of problems. For example, comfrey, which is an excellent wound-healing herb, can cause disastrous liver damage if taken internally. Therefore, make sure you're following the precise use of the remedy either internally or externally.

- **Know how and when to use essential oils:** Essential oils are oils taken directly from the plant, and as such, they are very aromatic and powerful. So, they should be used with care. If you're going to use the herbs externally, you should use them with a carrier oil.

  If you want to massage your partner's shoulders with essential oil, use only a few drops with a greater amount of coconut, olive, or sunflower oil, basically 1-part essential oil to 20 parts carrier oil. An essential oil should never be taken internally unless you are under the supervision of a doctor. This can have severe negative effects on your organs—and you kind of need those organs to function. So, take some care when using essential oils for herbal remedies.

- **Know the parts of the plant you're using:** Different parts of plants can have different effects; for example, the berries of the herbs pokeweed are toxic, but their leaves have been used for herbal remedies in the past. So, it's important to know which parts of the plant must be used. Aerial parts include leaves, stems, and flowers. Roots are, well, roots. So, know which part you should use for the safest effects.

- **Know what the plant looks like:** Mistaken identity can be a very costly error. You should know what each herb looks like before using it. You don't want to use a different herb that looks similar. This is just the case when foraging for mushrooms. Another example is how St. John's Wort is similar to ragweed, which is toxic. Knowing how to identify the herbs properly can help in ensuring that you are choosing the right one. This chapter doesn't talk about identifying herbs, but you can find many resources online for identifying herbs properly.

- **Know your prescriptions and how they may be affected by herbal remedies:** While most herbal remedies are useful when you are already taking medications, some of them can lessen the effectiveness of your prescriptions. If you are taking a prescription, talk to your doctor or herbalist about possible reactions between herbal remedies and your medication.

Dosages

Following the right dosage for each remedy is crucial to help you get better.

For the adult doses, follow their measurements and times precisely. Don't double remedies—just like you wouldn't double heart medication. Finally, don't take more than 2 herbal remedies at one time, as they may cancel each other out or cause more negative effects.

Some of the remedies mentioned here are useful for women who are pregnant, children, or the elderly, but the dosages need to change. Here are the changes to be made:

- For babies, don't give any herbal remedies if they're under the age of 6 months old.
- For a 6-month-old to a 1-year-old, give 1/10 of the adult dose, measured by weight.
- For a 1-year-old to a 6-year-old, give ⅓ of the adult dose, measured by weight.
- For a 7-year-old to a 12-year-old, give ½ of the adult dose, measured by weight.
- For elderly adults, give ¾ of the adult dose, measured by weight.
- For pregnant women in other trimesters, unless the remedy says it's safe for pregnant women, try not to take any herbal remedies unless prescribed by a doctor.

After taking the herbal remedy for 2–3 weeks, if you still don't see any improvement, see a doctor. If you see any negative effects, see a doctor. And, if you are seriously ill or wounded, you should, again, see a doctor.

The Active Substances in Herbs that Give Benefits to Body and Mind

Herbs have been a part of human culture for well over 50,000 years. Every culture across the globe has some form of herbal medicine tradition, and people use herbs for relief from physical and mental ailments.

We've put together this list of herbs to clarify which ones are best for what, including any warnings or precautions to take with them.

Herbal products are essentially plant-based remedies that can be taken orally or applied to the skin, but they all contain active substances derived from plants regardless of form, and those active substances in herbs give benefits to the body and mind.

Today, we are starting to learn more about how these herbs help us stay healthy. They are not only a part of many herbal product lines but herbalists and naturopaths also use them as remedies for a variety of ailments. Some herbs have even been found to boost the immune system, improve heart health, lower cholesterol, and act as stimulants for the body.

They have also helped in providing relief from stress and anxiety, which is a problem that many in society face, especially as our daily lives become more hectic and stressful. However, the benefits of herbs go beyond just treating your aches and pains or itches; they can also actively improve your day-to-day life in other ways.

This chapter will explore some popular herbs with their active substances that give benefits to the body and mind. Herbs have long been an essential part of natural health care. They are medicinal plants with a high therapeutic potential for treating illnesses.

Certain herbs have psychoactive properties that give benefits to the body and mind, which is one way they help people relax, relieve stress, or even get high. Different herbs contain different active substances. The amounts of the active substances vary between individuals and from one species to another. A healthy body can handle just a tiny number of active substances.

Some herbal medicines were used to cure illnesses like high blood pressure, and others as a natural alternative to over-the-counter treatments. Herbal remedies are now being studied in hospitals worldwide because they are becoming more and more critical. We will cover which herbs are traditionally used for, which active substances they contain, and how those substances benefit you physically and mentally.

Benefits of Using a Variety of Herbs

What are the benefits of adding a variety of herbs to your dietary intake?

There are many, but one significant advantage is that it promotes healthy bacteria in the gut. This is because all plants contain large amounts of polyphenols, which promote gut health by influencing these beneficial bacteria's population and activity. Herbs also contain many active substances that benefit the body and mind, including those with antidepressant properties like St John's wort and Valerian root.

All plants contain large amounts of polyphenols, which promote gut health by influencing beneficial bacteria's population and activity. The complex mixtures of polyphenols in plants are called "proanthocyanidins," which are highly water-soluble polymers containing between 600 and 2000 molecules per molecule.

Digestive enzymes break down "proanthocyanidins" into more minor elements with molecular weights between 5,000 and 10,000 that can be absorbed into the bloodstream. The more minor components are called "A-type proanthocyanidins" (A-PACs) and can extract minerals from water and other molecules. They can also bind chemicals in the body—such as heavy metals, bacterial endotoxins, and toxic environmental substances—and remove them from the colon.

Additionally, they have been found to stimulate the immune system, increase blood flow into inflamed joints by increasing small vessel diameter (dilating blood vessels), prevent platelets from clumping together in high blood pressure, thrombosis, and reduce clotting proteins.

The various plants used for medicinal purposes have one thing in common: They all contain multiple chemicals, known as "active substances." Some of those chemicals are poisonous, while others can be beneficial to us when consumed in appropriate quantities.

The active substances in herbs are the parts that give health benefits to our body and mind via their chemical compounds. These compounds can be tricky for our bodies and brains, so they have a complicated effect on people's emotions and behavior.

In general, the most common beneficial substances in herbs from which you get the most important benefits for the mind and body are:

Alkaloids

They are effective organic nitrogenous constituents for treating various diseases because they are capable of remarkable pharmacological effects.

Alkaloids include substances that act on the neuromuscular system, such as caffeine, morphine, nicotine, and mescaline. Given their exciting and depressing properties, alkaloids should be taken under strict medical supervision to avoid dangerous effects or interactions with other drugs. The plants richest in alkaloids are tea, coffee, tobacco, and in general, all plants belonging to the families of "Ranunculaceae," "Solanaceae," and poppies.

Polyphenols

They are powerful natural antioxidants able to combat cellular aging caused by free radicals. The polyphenols belong to tannins classified as "polyhydroxyphenol" compounds extracted from barks, roots, fruits, and leaves. They have an astringent action and are therefore indicated in treating injuries and wounds to promote tissue healing. Their use is also recommended to treat hemorrhoids and raghades. For internal use, they are used to fight diarrhea, enteritis, and inflammatory states in the intestine and gastric mucosa.

Flavonoids (or "Biflavonoids")

They are similar in characteristics to polyphenols because they perform identical antioxidant and coloring functions. Moreover, some flavonoids are obtained glycosides or substances responsible for storing sugars (ginseng, Echinacea, licorice, rhubarb, etc.).

Terpenes ("Terpenoids")

Characterize the essential oils most used in cosmetics; they are responsible for odors and scents of flowers and plants—just think of limonene, camphor, and menthol.

Starches

Derived from the transformation of sugar and characterized by a high degree of digestibility, starches are generally taken in synergy with other active ingredients and as a base for dietetic products.

Glycosides

They are chemical compounds consisting of a sugar group and a non-sugar group called "aglycone." Given the effect they have on the human body, their use is recommended under strict medical supervision. The main glucosides have important cardiotonic, anti-inflammatory, analgesic, diuretic, rheumatic, laxative, vasodilator, antispasmodic, antiseptic, and sweating functions. Some types of glucosides, if ingested in excessive doses, can be poisonous and cause cardiovascular arrest.

Mucilage

It is more than an active ingredient; mucilage is the result of a vegetative process.

In contact with water, they dilate and become dense and sticky. Their effectiveness is tested in treating the respiratory tract's inflammatory states, irritating the gastric and intestinal mucosa. Mallow and marshmallow are the plants richest in mucilage and are used in natural therapies to treat sore throat, pharyngitis, laryngitis, etc.

Essential Oils

Given their infinite beneficial properties, essential oils are among the substances of natural origin most used in phyto cosmetics and phytotherapy.

Essential oils generally stimulate the skin and mucous membranes, as well as the expectorant and fluidifying functions of the respiratory system. The plant's varieties richer in essential oils are those belonging to the families of "Labiatae" (mint and sage), "Pinaceae" (mountain pine), and "Umbelliferae" (aniseed and fennel).

I have also found four good reasons to treat yourself with herbs; if we use herbs and herbal remedies conscientiously, they can curb those minor ailments that afflict us during our everyday life. Mankind has always placed great trust and respect in nature, extracting both food and care from it, and over the millennia has selected and described all those herbal remedies that could help in healing or preventing certain diseases. Many of the latter, especially those of psychosomatic origin, can be cured effectively using only herbal extracts and medicinal plants and supplements.

Irritable bowel, constipation, dermatitis, headaches, gastritis, etc. whose cause is not an external pathogen (viruses, microbes, bacteria, etc.), but depends on our psyche, are often treated by the use of symptomatic drugs, which can soothe at the time but do not cure permanently this type of disorders. Therefore, over time, taking these synthetic remedies can cause intoxication or sensitization to their active ingredients.

Cure with Softness

From the curative point of view, when you take a plant, you do not benefit from the effect of a single active ingredient, as in the case of traditional medicines. Still, you use the synergistic action of a set of active ingredients in the drug's plant complex. This leads to the drastic reduction or total absence of side or undesirable effects (those reported on the package leaflets of medicines).

In the long term, especially for the above-mentioned psychosomatic diseases, the intake of medications consisting of a single active ingredient enhanced in the laboratory causes accumulation, sensitization, and intoxication of immune organs, such as liver, kidneys, and skin. On the other hand, plants act by their phyto complex's synergy, i.e., the active ingredients in it, which work together to produce a result not obtainable individually, modulating each other without causing side effects.

Moreover, as far as the assimilation is concerned, especially in the case of vitamins and mineral salts, when they are of vegetable origin, they are absorbed much better by our organism than those created and formulated in the laboratory. For example, the iron that comes from spirulina is immediately recognized and assimilated by our body because after being worked for itself by the seaweed, it returns it to us in a form immediately available.

Protect Animals

From an ethical perspective, natural products found in herbalists, especially cosmetics, are not tested on animals. This avoids unnecessary suffering and cruelty to animals due to vivisection. Moreover, a plant cannot be patented because it is a living being and not an invention unless it is genetically manipulated, and if this were the case, natural products would no longer be the field of phytotherapy but of genetic engineering and the pharmaceutical industry—which need to invent plants to be patented for economic reasons.

The herbalist, often using spontaneous plants, even if they found a very effective recipe, cannot patent it but remains confined to their herbal art's secrets and merges with their personal experience.

Do Not Pollute

The increase in the number of those who decide to take care of themselves with herbs leads to a more significant increase in the cultivation of medicinal plants in large geographical areas to meet the demand or maintain the pristine regions for those so-called spontaneous. Besides, natural cosmetics are free of foaming agents and other pollutants.

There is a plant for each of us from the individual's point of view, so, finally, taking care of herbs means rediscovering our individual uniqueness. The herbalist, when it is such, composes a custom blend concerning the indications that the customer reports. We are all different; we react to life in different ways, and our body manages even the disorders we suffer in different and utterly subjective manners. Going to an herbalist's shop means affirming all this and knowing that there is an appropriate remedy for each person.

Growing Your Own Herbs

The secret is starting small: Many plants are very easy to cultivate and can thrive even in a pot beside a sunny window in your city apartment. Among these plants, there are many that can be used for medical purposes, such as mint, thyme, or sage.

Before starting this adventure, be sure to go to your local extension office to test the quality of the soil with easy DYI (Define Your Inspiration) testing kits that cost about 10$.

These highly underrated offices often offer classes and advice about gardening for a very interesting price.

Although you may find the herbs you need for your preparations in the grocery store or herbal shop, my advice is to rely on local producers; they may be more expensive, but the quality is higher and generally worth the price.

When purchasing herbs, you must look at the key factors to determine the quality:

Soil

Ask where the herbs have been cultivated, and research that country's regulation regarding pollution. This task may seem complicated, but many big retailers already offer this certification of conformity in their products. If you are interested in urban farms, ask them if they use clean soil and if they have water filtration systems

Growing Practices

The aspects you have to take care of when inquiring about growing practices are:

Fertilizers

Fertilizers are natural or artificial substances that contain the chemical elements that your herbs and plants need to improve their growth and productiveness. They help in enhancing the fertility of the soil or in replacing the chemical elements that the soil has taken from previous crops.

Insect's Management

Most of the herbs you will end up using are worth growing yourself, and although proper wildcrafting is the best choice, it is quite time-consuming.

Benefits of Growing Medicinal Plants

Growing medicinal plants provides numerous benefits to humans and the environment. The following are some of the benefits of growing medicinal plants in your garden:

Herbal Medicinal as Foods

The food part, in some cases, differs from the therapeutic part; for instance, it's often the blackberry root bark that is being used for medicinal purposes. But in most cases, it's the edible part of the plants that we consume as food, balancing and toning the body while adding spices to our meals, like peppermint, ginger, fennel, and cayenne (a common digestive and circulatory system tonic).

We ought to integrate such herbs more regularly into our diets and discover their use in a more formal way when the need arises. For example, we could make an infusion of fennel to stimulate appetite or digestion or to treat colic.

Herbs could be used to prepare other foods with medicinal effects during the ancient periods. A variety of herbal plants, including berries, elderflowers, St. John's Wort, licorice, wintergreen, ginger, and yarrow, were used to flavor and to preserve ales and beers.

Vegetable oils and vinegar can be infused with herbs such as cayenne, garlic, and rosemary—and served in salad and other meals to improve our health. Mead, a fermented drink made from honey, has its medicinal values but could also be prepared with herbs like heather to boost its medicinal richness.

Herbs to Boost Insect Diversity

Experienced homesteaders are aware that the solution to managing insects isn't a process for killing them but allowing even more insect diversity, mainly by growing flowering plants all through the growing seasons.

Numerous common herbal medicines, such as Echinacea, yarrow, calendula, fennel, peppermint, and chamomile, are flowering plants and also have the value of providing food and shelter to the beneficiaries. Growing flowering plants and herbs is more effective at boosting our insect allies when integrated with the crops to be protected instead of planting them separately.

Herbs as Fertility Plants

Clever homesteaders are also aware that we can grow more of our soil fertility. Fortunately, a number of the best fertility plants also possess medicinal properties. Comfrey, used for healing broken bones and wounds, and nettle is rich in protein and could be used to "spark" a compost heap or as nutritive mulches. Yellow dock and dandelion are deep-rooted active collectors that mine mineral deposits from the sub-soil, offering them to more shallow-rooted crops.

Herbs as Fodder Crops

A large number of medicinal herbs and plants perform dual functions, providing dried fodder or fresh green for our livestock. I discovered that yellow duck and dandelion remain green deeper into winter's cold than other forage plans—I dig them up and feed them to my flocks. Oats could be used to feed livestock and also make an excellent nerve tonic. Either self-harvested or cut and fed green, my geese love comfrey.

Other Landscape or Ecological Uses

Willow and hawthorn may be cultivated as a living fence, as a windbreak, or for shade. They provide essential environmental benefits like wildlife, bird's shelter, moderation of the wind effects, heat, and loss of soil humidity to evaporation—in addition to their therapeutic values.

One of the best ways to make sure that you are harvesting what you want without confusing it with a potentially toxic look-alike is to grow it yourself. Growing your own herbs is also a great time-saver if you use a particular herb frequently to save you from hunting it down in the wild.

One of the easiest ways to start an herbal garden is to transplant herbs that you have found in the wild. This way, you can be sure that the herbs will grow well in your climate. It is important to understand the needs of the plant before attempting to grow it. There are many books about gardening, which can help you determine the type of soil, the sunlight and water requirements, and the cold hardiness of each plant.

What you decide to grow will depend on a few factors. If you're considering an outside garden, then you need to find out what will thrive in your climate.

If you can't get the answers you need from an online search, then call your local county extension service. You can find them by searching online or by calling a local university.

Once you know what herbs to grow, then you need to increase your chances of success by seeking out advice on the soil, sunlight, and other growth requirements.

Foraging and Reaping

Cultivating herbs at home is an enjoyable way to taste fresh flavors all year long. Besides, as the weather starts becoming cooler and the days get shorter, that means just one thing: Harvest season.

There are a few things you can keep in mind when cultivating plants, no matter what herb you're picking. Here's a realistic tip: Just pick herbs when they're dry. It is advisable to reap after the morning dew has gone or at night.

Just before the buds open, you should harvest culinary herbs. Be sure to pinch several buds before they open since after they flower, all the plant's energy goes into developing blooms, and then the tasty leaves do not grow well.

Harvest the seeds until they turn from green to brown. The seeds have to be fragile, dry, and crushable.

Be gentle. Handle them carefully to stop bruising your precious crop when harvesting, as fresh herbs are fragile.

Sustainable Foraging Recommendations

1. The abundant plants with a broad, scattered population are forage only. Not extracting a plant for commercial demand without considering the loss of habitat, may pose to the plant population. For example, a plant may be geographically abundant, but if there is a universal ultimatum, it may easily disappear, with over-harvesting decimating the population.

2. Favor for harvesting nonnative species. If the herb is native and connected to local food chains or is a deserter from another location, it is among the first things we remember when choosing which herbs to eat. By competing with them for natural resources, nonnatives relocate native animals. With the same balances and checks that natural plants have encountered, these resourceful plants have not grown nearby, and so they often thrive. This brands them as primary forage for us humans, especially because they remain close to places we live, growing in neighborhoods, gardens, fields, and the like. Nonnatives include multiflora rose ("Rosa multiflora"), Japanese honeysuckle ("Lonicera japonica"), Mimosa ("Albizia julibrissin"), and burdock ("Arctium minus"). Several species of raspberry and blackberry ("Rubus spp") are some of our most popular wild feeble medicinal items in the United States (southeast).

3. Tend the gaps "in-between." Wild weeds will naturally arise and make themselves at home with those of you who cultivate a greenhouse and cohabit comfortably with developed vegetables and herbs. You can use plenty of techniques to make them play fair, and you can collect still more medication and food from your greenhouse as an opportunity to serve as a botanical referee! This is the bounty that develops between the medicines and vegetables you have not created yet or the ones you still have to reap. Frank Cook, a plant friend who died, used to teach in classes that, in the form of useful opportunistic plants, more than half of the abundance of a garden may be found in the "in-between."

People around the world profit from this vast resource, casually "cultivating" weeds in the regions in between.

Let us take the lamb's quarters as an example of this form of useful-weed-and-planted-crop polyculture. More protein, beta-carotene, vitamin C, zinc, and calcium than cultivated spinach are given by lamb parts, often called "wild spinach." Why will you root out such a strong plant that does not need special treatment or protection from pests to make way for crops that are less stable and more difficult to develop? You should leave the wild spinach in the field between the newly planted vegetables and the herbal crops. The vegetables fill up after planting the wild spinach for a few weeks or a month, and then you can take out the lamb's quarters and use them as mulch for the cultivated crops. Because it makes its way into the greenhouse, wild spinach needs little planting and is relatively disease-free and insect-free.

Be a steward purely, and when you pick sufficiently (possibly pesky) species, adhere to a code of ethics. You deal with, after all, real, breathing animals. Take what you need, leave the beauty of the wake (leave no trace), make a bid before you go, make a poem, a little water, hair, and a handful of grain. An offering demands a sense of appreciation, reciprocity, and respect.

If you are more science-minded, you might take a minute to consciously relax, meditating on the reciprocity of the exchange of plant-human oxygen, cellular respiration, and photosynthesis. At first, you can sound ridiculous, but give yourself the chance to be shocked. This is how the ancient plant-human dance of friendly touch, love and influences us.

Be very careful not to overharvest if the plant you are harvesting is organic, so you have already assessed that it is enough to produce. If you are picking a multi-stem herbaceous plant, cut out a stem or two from each plant.

Scatter the crop around a wider field and ensure that you leave the plants with enough flowers and fruit to reproduce. Replant the root crown while you are extracting roots or take only part of the root system of each plant.

Be careful to cut back the aboveground portions while digging up roots so that the plant does not get saturated by water with a root structure that no longer suits its aboveground growth. For resistant weeds with global dispersion, the SES regenerative methods do not even need to be pursued. Harvest in situations where you realize that no one has applied herbicide.

Since the surrounding soil is typically polluted with lead, herbicides, and other toxins, there should be no planting of plants near highways, railroads, and power lines. Typically, farm at least 30 feet from the road and make sure you do not farm in an environmentally sensitive area (such as a dirty river flood bank). Herbicides can be added in hay fields.

Wildcrafting

Wild crafting is the ancient art of harvesting untouched, natural growth areas of herbs and plants. Make sure you have permission to select and that normal outdoor security procedures are observed. When you harvest into the near future, make sure to take just what you will need; this will allow for enough growth in exchange for your next visit.

It is necessary that it be carried out with reverence and consciousness when one enters the world and the plants to obtain drugs. People who religiously receive medicine from Indigenous cultures have done so in identical ways around the globe. The behavioral patterns that underlie them remain the same, although some of the strategies can vary. It is only when plants are used as resources that they continue to be cultivated without thinking.

It can take months or even years to gain an appreciation of what you see when you walk into the plant environment. The experience of waking up early in the morning, hiking into the wild, and harvesting your own herbs is for sure a satisfactory one.

Sometimes this is not your best choice: Over-harvesting endangered plants or destroying the habitat of plants are big problems nowadays. You can easily check the list of endangered species on "unitedplantsaver.org."

If unsure, harvest no more than 10% native whole plants and roots and 30% naturalized plant species or native leaves and flowers. Gather only from abundant stands. Harvest conservatively to ensure the maintenance and well-being of plant communities.

Be Able to Identify Herbs

The first rule of wildcrafting is knowing what you're looking at. In other words, you need to be proficient at identifying plants and not just herbs.

You should have a rudimentary knowledge of weeds, bushes, and trees. You should learn how to spot a plant by its leaves and by the appearance of its fruit or berries.

This is the first rule because you don't want to harvest a dangerous doppelganger plant unaware. At best, using it could lead to mild discomfort. At worst, it could kill you.

Site Selection and Permission

On BLM land, a free use permit may be obtained for a minimal charge if you are collecting small amounts.

Stay away from downwind pollution, roadsides (at least 50 feet), high-tension electric wires (may cause mutations), fertilizers in lawns and public parks, downstream from mining or agribusiness, around parking lots, and possible sprayed areas. Some BLM and Forest Service districts use routine spraying.

This applies to private land as well, and you may need to ask about herbicides and pesticides.

Use discretion with fragile environments—one irresponsible wildcrafter can severely alter a rocky hillside or streamside ecosystem.

Gardening and Propagation Techniques

Be aware of erosion factors. If digging roots, replant or scatter the seeds and cover the holes. Be mindful of hillside stands; replace foliage and dirt around harvested areas. Gathering foliage from nearby harvested plants and spreading it around may be necessary. Wearing hard-soled shoes may cause delicate hillside ecosystems irreparable damage.

If harvesting leaf, don't pull the roots. Flower pruning of certain plants will increase root yields as well as foliage.

Make seasonal observations on wildcrafted areas. Be mindful of your harvested stands and check different growth cycles. This will determine your real impact on the ecosystem. (One experienced wildcrafter in the northwest has observed that a healthy population will increase about 30% a year until it reaches stasis. Anything less than this could be considered degenerative.)

Suggested Gathering Times

- **Aerial or Above-Ground Parts:** It is good to gather them in the mornings between 6 and 10 a.m., just before they wilt in the sun. If harvesting a leaf, many are best just before flowering.
  Harvest most flowers just as they are beginning to bloom—you should be able to see the color of the bud. The traditional moon phase for harvesting aerial parts is near or during the full moon.
- **Roots:** Harvest roots after seeding, if possible, in the early morning before the sun hits.
- **Biennials:** Harvest in the fall of the first year or the spring of the second year. The traditional phase is the new moon.
- **Barks:** Harvest in the spring or fall. Never strip. Take the whole tree. Tree thinning is appropriate in dense populations but always leaves the healthiest-looking trees, though. If you take from the small branches only, be aware of potentially leaving the tree vulnerable to fungal rot. For many barks, the inner bark, or cambium, is the most active. Leave short trunks for pollarding and low stumps for coppicing. This will provide an ongoing harvest. The traditional phase for barks is the three-quarter waning moon.
- **Saps and Pitches:** Harvest in late winter or early spring.
- **Seed and Fruit:** Harvest when mature, with some exceptions such as citrus, unripe scarlet bean pods, etc.

Foraging or an herb garden? Does this choice tear you? Don't be; because you can do both quite easily. An herb garden provides you with the ease of accessibility to your most used herbs, that daily one for distressing, healing injuries, or alleviating your daily aches and pains.

Just because you grow your own herbs doesn't mean you can't go on an occasional foraging adventure. Foraging, which is nothing more than discovering and harvesting plants in the wild, doesn't have to be intimidating. It can be as simple as going into a meadow and searching for clovers or daisies.

When you forage for your herbs, you're wildcrafting. It's the process of gathering herbs in their natural environment. The herbs or dried herbs you buy from stores, even health food stores, were not grown in their natural environment unless explicitly indicated on the packaging. Besides, many herbalists believe responsible wildcrafting has two advantages.

The first is that the herbs are more powerful when grown in their natural environment. Instead of being bred for sale, these herbs are receiving nutrients from the soil naturally. Getting nutrients through natural means is also better for your health and well-being.

The other advantage, though, involves your relationship with Mother Nature. It's something Grace would tell me, "Wildcrafting for the herbs you need at the moment and no more ruining humanity's relationship with nature." As you forage, you'll look upon these plants as friends and allies in your healing, not merely as a product to be used.

Because Grace saw herbs this way, she always asked permission of the plant before harvesting it. This concept sounds wild and woo-woo to many westerners, but the best wildcrafters practice this courtesy even today.

It may take you some time before you feel the connection with the plant world that Grace did, but it's there. It took me some months of wildcrafting with my friend before I felt that connection. At first, it seemed slight and far away, but as I spent more time with the plants, the relationships grew.

Bring the Proper Tools

Prepare for your excursion, even if you only plan to spend a short time.

You'll want to take with you either a pair of scissors or a pocket knife. I know some herbalists take a pair of small pruning shears if they are searching for larger plants. The cutting tools you take will depend on your potential harvest. But if you find an herb you weren't searching for but think will help you, you may want to carry a variety of tools.

Whatever you do, don't tear or rip the plant. You'll want the clean cut of a utensil. For one thing, a clean cut will help spur new growth. The purpose of wildcrafting is to preserve the environment. Ripping parts of plants defeats that purpose.

If you're foraging for roots, then don't forget to pack a small gardener's trowel. If you're going to be gone for long, then instead of taking a basket, you may want to take a box of sandwich-size plastic bags for temporary storage.

And lastly, always include a bottle of water and perhaps some snacks, and don't forget a small first-aid kit.

Harvest with Permission

While you need the plant's permission, you also need the consent of the owner of the private land. Before you go, research the area you plan on harvesting from. If it's private, check with the owner before embarking. If it's federal land, be sure harvesting is allowed.

Harvest with the Welfare of the Plants in Mind

When you harvest parts from any group of plants, you should never take more than 20% of them. That's what responsible wildcrafting is all about. If you take more than that percentage, the odds increase that the plants can be damaged or be placed in shock, or they may even die. If there are five plants, only take what would be 20% of a plant. This may mean taking a leaf from several herbs instead of depleting an entire plant.

The concept behind this is harvesting to the needs of the plants. While foraging, consider what the plant or the community of plants needs to live. Don't take so much as to destroy the plant or injure the plant community.

You will also want to look around at where they're growing. If you find an invasive weed that you know will damage the plants, remove it for them. If there are broken branches around that may impede their growth, so remove them as well. The plants will appreciate it.

Walk Deliberately

You're not in a race. In fact, you're in whatever the opposite of a race is.

Tread lightly. Don't walk on herbs wantonly; make your way with care so as to disturb the area as little as possible. While you're walking with a light step, keep your eyes lowered. Be aware of plants that may be hidden by other larger shrubs or covering.

At times, you'll just stop; that's right. Take a good look around, not only for the plants but to enjoy your surroundings.

Methods to Become an Expert Herbalist

Dried herbs are also used in teas (also known as tisanes, a lovely French term), infusions, or decoctions. The difference among different teas is the volume of dry plant material used in comparison to the amount of water used, as well as the length of time it is steeped or simmered. It is not to be confused with black tea, such as Darjeeling or oolong, which has its own cult.

Aluminum and iron can never be used to make remedies since they have a negative reaction to the plants.

Instead, cook your brews with stainless steel, enamelware, or heat-tempered glass, and use good water. You may want to invest in a water filter for your daily drinking water if you have chlorinated municipal water.

Herbal Tea

Use 1 rounded tsp. (not exactly a measuring teaspoon, but the sort you stir with) of dried, crushed plant material or 2 teaspoons of fresh plant material to a teacup or mug full of boiling water for a basic herbal beverage or tisane. Steep it (soak) for just a few minutes.

To make it simpler to strain, soak it in a jar or teapot, then spill it into a cup and sweeten it if necessary. While most teas are diuretic to a degree, 2 or 3 cups a day is not excessive.

Tea can be made from a variety of spices, such as spearmint, chamomile, or nettles, and it's pleasant to try different flavor variations.

Herbal Infusion

A strong tea used as a medicine is known as an "herbal infusion." Add one ounce of dry plant material (usually leaves or flowers) to one pint of boiling water, cover, and steep for 10 to 15 minutes. The herb is not cooked in either way.

Remove the strainer and serve. This is the herbal tea dosage, and depending on the cure, you can only take a couple of sips at a time. Some guidelines specify whether to drink hot or cold, as well as the right time of day to drink.

Herbal Decoction

Use 1 ounce of dry plant material (usually a harder part of the plant, such as the base, bark, twig, seed, or berry) to 1 pint of water for a decoction, and then add a good herbal tea that is simmered. Cover and boil for around 15 minutes, depending on the plant parts and desired weight. In realistic terms, an ounce of dry plant material will hold up to a cup of liquid.

Herbal Poultice, or Plaster

The curing operation of this process of utilizing herbs is aided by the use of moisture and heat. They're used to treat wounds, minimize pain, break up congestion, and function as a sliver or infection-drawing agent.

Simple Poultice

Fresh herbs, such as chickweed, self-heal (heal-all), violet leaf, or other gentle emollient herbs, maybe mashed up in a bowl with a fork or a wooden spoon, buzzed in a blender, or chewed into a pulp (this is particularly useful out on the trail) and applied directly to the infected region is one way to create a poultice — the simplest way, in truth.

The poultice is held in place with a slice of cabbage, plantain, or another broad, non-irritating leaf tightly protected with a strip of gauze ribbon.

Alternatively, you should just stay still for a couple of minutes while the poultice does its magic and then go about your business. Chickweed (Stellaria media), a native garden "weed," may be used to treat contaminated splinters.

Compound Plaster

Another kind of poultice, or plaster, is produced by grinding the desired dried herb, combining it with an equivalent amount of bran, oatmeal, or flaxseed meal (or another neutral medium), and then adding only enough very hot water to create a wet paste.

The quantities required are determined by the size of the area to be covered. Cover with a soft, moistened piece of muslin or a piece of cheesecloth designed to fit over the infected region, then cover with a dry cloth. A common Chinese treatment for pulmonary problems, such as the chest, kidney blockage, middle back, and menstrual cramps, is a ginger compress (abdomen and lower back).

The herbal plaster is less common than a plain poultice or herb compress, partly because it is more expensive and partly because it is challenging to spread on one's own. Some plasters, such as plaster apples for sunburn, may be produced without the bran and just the plant material.

Herb Compress

A compress is equivalent to plaster, but it is often less complicated to use. A solid, hot infusion of the herb of choice is produced.

Dip soft cloths or towels in the tea, wring them out, and then apply to the infected region. Cover the "user" with a towel or blanket to keep them covered.

Any compresses, such as those for sunburn or sprains, can be cool. Of course, certain cases, such as a fractured bone, will necessitate the usage of cold applications, at least before immediate medical help arrives. We must use justification and common sense while handling ourselves, and understanding our limits is part of it.

Herbal Tinctures

A way of concentrating the therapeutic properties of herbs for internal usage is to make an alcohol-based tincture with fresh or dried herbs. Herbal tinctures have the advantage of lasting almost indefinitely.

These are made by steeping one pint (or sufficient liquid to cover the herb) of good-quality vodka in a new, clean jar with approximately 1 ounce of dried or 4 ounces of fresh plant material, chopped or gently crushed (do not powder).

Put the date and label it. The tincture can steep for 2 weeks or longer if the compound is thicker. Although certain herbalists recommend brandy or gin for certain fresh flowers, leaves, and dried plants, we choose vodka (which is precisely 50% alcohol and 50% water).

For fresh roots or other rugged or resinous plant stuff, such as cottonwood buds, pure grain alcohol, or Everclear®, is highly recommended; if you can't find Everclear®, consider 151® proof rum.

Since tinctures are condensed, the dosage is normally given in drops (rather than droppers-full), ranging between 10 to 30 drops per adult dose, depending on the herbs and the person's weight. To avoid burning your tongue, dilute the drops in the water.

Rubbing alcohol and wood alcohol can never be used internally since they are highly harmful once consumed. You may produce an herbal liniment for exterior use with rubbing alcohol, but good old vodka is recommended for this.

Well, it is more costly, but it is also better. Fill small dropper bottles of your tinctures, which you can get from your nearest pharmacy or buy online. Mark all of your herbal items with the date, ingredients, and intended use.

Herbal Wine

Certain herbs may be steeped in wine; for example, May® wine, which is made with sweet woodruff and German white wine, but these are meant to be consumed right away since they don't keep well.

You know if they're a good way to take your medication or a medicinal way to enjoy your enjoyment. To infuse the wine with herbs, pour one bottle (1 quarter, 45 quarts, or 750 ml) of wine into a quart jar with a half cup of fresh, clean herbs or edible flowers — the combinations of which are only limited by your imagination.

If you're using dried spices like clove or cinnamon, just use a few bits at a time because they're very potent.

The elder steal, which is made from dried elderberries and a cinnamon stick mulled over a dry red wine like burgundy, is one example of herb-infused wine for medicinal purposes.

Infusing herbs in wine solely for flavoring purposes is perfectly acceptable.

Oil Extracts

To render soothing rubs for a variety of uses, soak such herbs in oil.

Pure olive oil has a long shelf life and is the most often used oil for salves — almond oil makes a fine basis for special body oils.

Place 1 pint of oil, 2 ounces of dried plant material, or 4 ounces of fresh herbs in a small saucepan, and cover it with more oil if desired.

Place the saucepan over a low heat setting and soak the herbs in the oil for many hours, stirring regularly to avoid scorching. You will want to steep for a couple of days depending on the plant material; in this situation, switch off the heat overnight (cover with a towel so it can still evaporate) and restart the gentle heat in the morning.

When the oil smells fragrant and has a rich color from the herbs — indeed, the herbs may have lost some of their green colors — it is primed. After straining out the herbs, cool the oil slightly before placing it in a clean, dry container.

It has been discovered that a mini slow cooker is an excellent gentle warming vessel for steeping herbs in oil, especially fresh herbs since you can leave the lid off to allow the water in the plant material to evaporate and keep it running for a couple of days without concern.

The herbs can mold if you don't use some heat and instead soak fresh herbs and oil in a container with the lid on. As a result, unless vinegar is used, it is no longer advisable to infuse garlic in oil for any amount of time, as it may trigger botulism in an anaerobic (airless) atmosphere. While you are unlikely to use herbal oil extracts, the idea remains the same.

While you're using fresh plants, gentle heat of any kind is recommended.

Herbal oil extracted from birch twigs or cottonwood buds produces a wonderful analgesic rub that often smells great.

For bruising and muscle spasms, apply St. John's Wort spray. Make an after-shower body oil by steeping fragrant flower petals and herbs. Glass bottles are best for storing oils.

Herbal Salves, Ointments, Balms, and Unguents

What do you owe a sore throated pig? Ointment! Anyway, these words are synonymous and apply to treatments for superficial scrapes, abrasions, and a variety of skin ailments.

They are oil extracts prepared as before and thickened or hardened with beeswax or another strong fat, such as cocoa butter or coconut oil, or made deer tallow if you have a hunter in the home. "Lip balm" is really a fancy word for "salve."

Make the salve with herbs that fit your needs, such as cedar leaves for antifungal properties, chickweed, and plantain for emollient properties, Oregon grape leaf for infection prevention, or comfrey root for rapid healing.

Basic Salve

Stir approximately 1 ounce of grated beeswax into 1 pint of warm oil extract prepared as directed above. You'll have to experiment if you're using a certain kind of thickener because it's difficult to predict how viscous the oil would be.

Scoop up a teaspoon of the oil-wax mixture and dump it onto a small plate to search its hardness; after a few minutes, it will have cooled, and you may measure its strength. It can slosh around in the bottle if it is too smooth, and it will be impossible to get a lick out of it if it is too stiff.

Salves may be formulated from several types of oil extracts or oil extracts made from a variety of herbs. Tiny quantities of other additives, such as honey, lanolin, or vitamin E oil, may also be added.

Put the label and date. Keep your salves in thin, wide-mouthed pots, but don't cover them until they're completely cool. Look for beautiful jars to offer as gifts.

Making salves is an organic, hands-on method that can be a little messy at times, but that's just part of the fun. Children may assist in the project by assisting in the identification and harvesting of medicinal plants.

Conclusion

Native American herbalists and healers have used traditional plants for centuries, which are used all over the world. In fact, some of these plants are so popular that they've become global commercial crops.

Native American herbal practices involved a wide variety of plants and medicines, with certain Indian tribes in the Southwest and Pacific Northwest using many different types of plant materials to create the treatments that were most effective for their communities.

One thing you should remember is that most herbals are only effective when they come from a plant harvested from nature or grown in garden beds by an individual who understands its properties and uses it correctly. Similarly, Native Americans used the natural resources and properties of their surroundings to create remedies.

Native Americans used plants for a variety of reasons, including medical purposes. For example, the Navajo were known to use particular plants for improving the taste of mescal (a type of liquor created from the agave plant) and other herbs. Many Native Americans used various plants for medicinal purposes, such as the Apache, who used several plants for treating skin ailments. Today, Native Americans may still use traditional herbal treatments in similar ways if they choose to do so. Herbal knowledge was passed down from generation to generation, and the most commonly used plants were well known by the people who knew them well.

The traditional healing practices of the Native Americans were also used as a guide for modern western medicine. Many Westerners utilize these practices as a complementary aid to the modern pharmacological approaches practiced by doctors, which include the use of pharmaceutical and natural ingredients. These herbal remedies may be taken by mouth, massaged into the skin, or used topically, such as in baths or oils.

In many cases, Native American medicinal plants were considered sacred and held in high regard by Native communities who collected them with great care. They were often mixed with animal parts, minerals, or other plant materials, perhaps as a means of increasing their potency.

The use of medicinal plants was practiced within other societies in Asia and the Americas. While many Native American medicinal plants are still used in modern herbal medicine, others have declined in popularity or use due to the rise of modern medical practices and the availability of synthetic drugs.

Since the mid-20th century, some Native Americans have become increasingly involved in assimilating Western medicine into their culture by opening hospitals and clinics, which are staffed by both Native American healers and "conventional" medical doctors trained in mainstream Western schools. Such contemporary practices include the use of medicinal plants to treat a variety of conditions, including diabetes, infections, and inflammation.

The Native American herbal tradition is actually one of the oldest traditions in all of human history. Because Native American culture has existed for thousands of years, their medicinal plants were continuously passed on from generation to generation. As a result, contemporary herbal remedies used today by Native Americans have been adapted to utilize Western herbs and are often mixed with other natural materials.

Native American herbal remedies are mostly gathered from plants and herbs that grow wild. They would make infusions, decoctions, tinctures, poultices, or ointments with these plants.

A big reason they used herbal remedies was that they did not have access to modern medicines at the time due to the harsh environment.

Today, you can take advantage of these traditional remedies too by choosing to incorporate herbal healing into your life. The use of herbs in natural medicine is one of the most holistic forms of healing available today.

Glossary

Ginger has been used in traditional Chinese medicine for years to treat muscle pain and other body pains that come with aging. 104

Ginger Root: The ginger plant is a perennial climbing herb that produces rhizomes and roots. It grows on other plants and can grow up to as high as 1.5 meters with lush green leaves that are spotted with reddish or yellowish-brown spots. 105

Goldenseal: Find a tincture or glycerin extract (it's a lot more concentrated) and use this herb to help with "hot flashes" associated with menopause. It is also used for purification (like sage). 111

Green tea is another popular herbal supplement, with numerous reports of it being effective for weight loss and the prevention of many cancers 118

Hibiscus Tea: The hibiscus flower has been used for numerous health treatments. 106

is a plant of the family of Composites. In Italy, depending on the place, it is known by the names of amarella, amareggiola, matricale, maresina and marga grass. 94

Kava Kava: The root is used in ceremonies. It aids in purification by effectively "clearing" a space of negative influences. 111

Lavender: The flowers are used for relaxation, protection from negative energy (like a sage), and fertility. 108

Lemon Balm: This plant contains numerous essential oils that have been used in medicinal treatments for centuries, most commonly for headaches. 106

Licorice is the root of a plant and can be found in tea, candy, gum, and even cough drops 101

Lotus has a spiritual energy that helps one rest in peace within herself or himself; a symbol of purity, self-love, and self-acceptance which is essential for prosperity in all aspects of life. 102

Marigold is symbolic of abundance in all areas of life; it relates to financial prosperity. Used in ceremonies for banishing evil spirits from the home or business environment. 102

Mind/Body Medicine - using holistic practices with herbal remedies or practices which help clear up physical ailments through mental guidance without prescription drugs 125

Mint is one of the most popular herbs today. It can be found in candies, gum, toothpaste, and many dishes like lamb chops 101

Mugwort: A powerful purifier of negative energy (like sage). 109

Mullein has been used to alleviate pain and fever associated with sickness or injuries 102

one of the most present vegetables on the tables of the Mediterranean area. 93

Patchouli is spicy and grounding. It helps with protection from evil spirits and attracts good fortune in business ventures. 102

Praying Medicine - using certain substances to heal a person of disease or illness through prayer 125

Rosemary is stimulating and strengthening the mind. It helps with blood circulation, in memory, and focus. 102

Sage is warming and vibrant. It helps with nerve pain, headaches, and muscle aches. 102

Sage: Both leaves and flowers are used to carry negativity away, protect from negative spirits, and cleanse your aura 110

Spiritual Healing - performing rituals such as sweat lodges or fire cleansings to migrate spiritual energy in order to bring balance in all aspects of life 125

Sumac is excellent for treating colds, fevers and sore throats. 98

The composition of black raspberries cannot be compared to the composition of red berries or blackberries. A lot of precious substances included. 80

The drug consists of the flowering tops of Achillea M. millefolium 69

The drug is the secondary roots of Harpagophytum procumbens (Burch) DC. (fam. Pedaliaceae), a herbaceous plant that grows wild in the Kalahari desert. The name of the genus comes from the Greek 73

The elderflower extract is what is used for medicinal purposes. 93

The pollen derives its name from the Latin pollen, or fior di farina. It is in fact presented as a powder of variable color (yellow-red). 74

Thyme is cleansing and sweet. It helps with fear of success or failure, fear of change, anxiety as well as insomnia. 102

Traditional Healing - wordless chants that include visualization of a vision or a plant 125

Turmeric is used to cleanse the home or business environment from evil spirits or negative energies. 102

Valerian helps to calm down the nerves. This amazing herb has been proven to be effective in treating insomnia by inducing lucid dreams.
White Windsor: The leaves are used for purification and protection from negativity (like a sage).

References

Herbal Medicine. (n.d.). Johns Hopkins Medicine. Retrieved August 15, 2021, from https://www.hopkinsmedicine.org/health/wellness-and-prevention/herbal-medicine

Healing Plants—Medicine Ways: Traditional Healers and Healing—Healing Ways—Exhibition—Native Voices. (n.d.). Native Voices. Retrieved August 13, 2021, from https://www.nlm.nih.gov/nativevoices/exhibition/healing-ways/medicine-ways/healing-plants.html

Herbal medicine—Better Health Channel. (n.d.). Better Health Channel. Retrieved August 15, 2021, from https://www.betterhealth.vic.gov.au/health/conditionsandtreatments/herbal-medicine

How Do Herbs Work? An Introduction to Herbal Modes of Action and Use—WSAVA 2015 Congress—VIN. (n.d.). VIN. Retrieved August 15, 2021, from https://www.vin.com/apputil/content/defaultadv1.aspx?id=7259347&pid=14365&print=1

http://www.jcreview.com/fulltext/197-1580283855.pdf?1580292874. (2020). Journal of Critical Reviews, 7(01). https://doi.org/10.31838/jcr.07.01.57

How Should Allopathic Physicians Respond to Native American Patients Hesitant About Allopathic Medicine? (2020). AMA Journal of Ethics, 22(10), E837-844. https://doi.org/10.1001/amajethics.2020.837

Encapsulated Indian medicinal herb shows anti-diabetic properties in mice. (n.d.). Science Daily. Retrieved August 15, 2021, from https://www.sciencedaily.com/releases/2019/07/190731113017.htm

Encyclopedia of Herbal Medicine. (n.d.). Google Books. Retrieved August 13, 2021, from https://books.google.com.ph/books/about/Encyclopedia_of_Herbal_Medicine.html?id=3MbaDwAAQBAJ&printsec=frontcover&source=kp_read_button&hl=en&redir_esc=y#v=onepage&q&f=false

14 Amazing Natural Herbs to Attract Wealth and Prosperity! (n.d.). Longevity. Retrieved August 13, 2021, from https://vocal.media/longevity/14-amazing-natural-herbs-to-attract-wealth-and-prosperity

Deering, S. (2019, February 28). Nature's 9 Most Powerful Medicinal Plants and the Science Behind Them. Healthline. https://www.healthline.com/health/most-powerful-medicinal-plants

Ozioma, E. J. (2019, January 30). Herbal Medicines in African Traditional Medicine. IntechOpen. https://www.intechopen.com/chapters/64851

The Healthline Editorial Team. (2018, September 18). Homegrown Herbal Remedies. Healthline. https://www.healthline.com/health/herbal-remedies-from-your-garden

Pollux, A. (2021, February 14). Our 9 Favourite Magickal Herbs for Love. Welcome To Wicca Now. https://wiccanow.com/herbs-for-love/

Herbs and Spices. (2019, October 1). College of Agricultural Sciences. https://horticulture.oregonstate.edu/oregon-vegetables/herbs-and-spices-0

Native and Indigenous Communities and Mental Health. (n.d.). Mental Health America. Retrieved August 13, 2021, from https://www.mhanational.org/issues/native-and-indigenous-communities-and-mental-health

Burgess, L. (2019, February 28). 12 natural ways to relieve pain. Medical News Today. https://www.medicalnewstoday.com/articles/324572

Cherney, K. (2020, June 1). 9 Herbs to Fight Arthritis Pain. Healthline. https://www.healthline.com/health/osteoarthritis/herbs-arthritis-pain

Healing Plants - Medicine Ways: Traditional Healers and Healing - Healing Ways - Exhibition - Native Voices. (n.d.). Native Voices. Retrieved August 13, 2021, from https://www.nlm.nih.gov/nativevoices/exhibition/healing-ways/medicine-ways/healing-plants.html

MDLinx International. (n.d.). MDLinx International. Retrieved August 13, 2021, from https://www.mdlinx.com/article/9-clinically-proven-natural-remedies-for-common-ailments/2pwhB5S2HywOusXbWIDbHF